THE DENTAL CONNECTION

The Role of Holistic Dentistry
in the Integrative Healing Paradigm

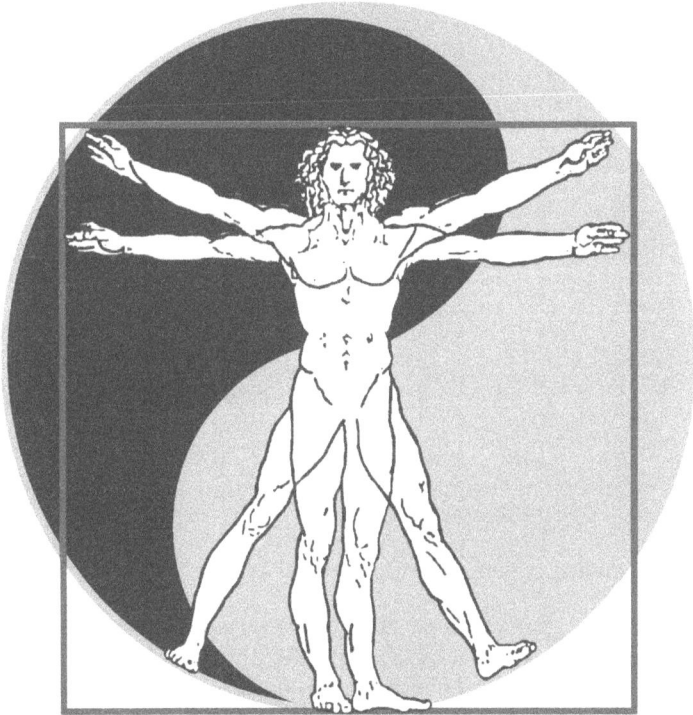

David L. Lerner, D.D.S., C.Ac., L.V.I.F.

*Thanks to my beloved wife Marisa and our daughter Donielle
for their love, patience, and dedication.*

To my team without whom I couldn't get much done.

*To my mentors and teachers and those
who came before us who showed us the way.*

*And to the thousands of patients I have cared for over the years
who taught me so much.*

TABLE OF CONTENTS

PREFACE
My Story

My evolution as a holistic dentist really began way before I had thought of becoming a dentist. It began when I was a kid. When I was going to the dentist, I always had lots of cavities. It seemed that with every checkup, there were more mercury silver fillings to be placed. Then I needed braces. Because I had lost a tooth (a premolar) in my lower jaw due to an accident, the orthodontist decided to close the space by bringing my teeth all the way over across the front, from the right to the left. My teeth ended up looking straight, but my jaw was crooked.

I had a difficult time in school. Everyone told me I was an underachiever. (Today they might have recognized that I had a learning disability.) I had difficulty processing information that I would read—a form of dyslexia. I also had a difficult time with sports because I had poor coordination. I always had headaches and assumed that everyone did. Years later, I was to discover that this all had a lot to do with the conditions in my mouth and how the rest of my body was being influenced by it.

Subsequent to my graduation with honors from Temple University School of Dentistry in 1978, my headaches got worse and I developed neck discomfort. Though I often had headaches as a kid, this was worse. It turned out to be related to the misalignment of my jaw. In the summer of 1980, I got a biteplate and some physical therapy, and all seemed okay. My treating doctor was Dr. Richard Pertes who was head of the Department of Craniofacial Pain at the New Jersey School of Dentistry and Medicine. Dick introduced me to Dr. Harold Gelb, a pioneer in the multidisciplinary treatment of temporomandibular disorders. I was fortunate to work in Dr. Gelb's office as an associate for eighteen months.

During that time, my wife and I were living in Ossining, New York. One winter, there was a pretty good snowstorm, and being newlyweds, we had not yet acquired all the accoutrements of a suburban household and did not have a snow shovel. Well, my car needed to be dug out of the snow. All I could find was a frying pan, and so it went.

I injured my back, causing a subluxation between my lower lumbar spine and my sacrum. I was in pain! What made matters worse was I could not find a practitioner who knew how to treat me. I saw chiropractors, physicians, and physical therapists, but no one could provide any relief. As time when on, the pain got worse and spread over more of my body. Eventually, I had pain in my jaw, face, head, neck, and upper and lower back. I had pain shooting down my leg. It didn't matter if I stood, sat, or laid down, the pain was unrelenting and wore me down.

Eventually, I found Dr. Harold Briks, a chiropractor par excellence. Dr. Briks was an expert in the use of Applied Kinesiology and Sacral-Occipital Technique. Applied Kinesiology is a biofeedback technique that uses the phenomenon of muscle reflex testing discovered by Dr. George Goodheart back in the mid-60s. It allows a practitioner to diagnose disorders of the musculoskeletal system with great efficiency and precision. Sacral-Occipital Technique is a method of analysis and treatment of imbalances of the skull and sacrum developed by Dr. Major Dejarnette. These are discussed in more depth later on. From that very first visit with Dr. Briks, I started to experience relief. I was intrigued by his technique because with it, he would get great results for me. I started to attend chiropractic seminars on Applied Kinesiology and to study how to apply it in my dental practice.

Though I was getting great pain relief, I still wasn't feeling quite right and began to look elsewhere for additional answers. I experienced fatigue and had poor digestion. I went to a dentist named Bob Poritsky, DDS, who I knew practiced nutritional therapy. Bob was studying an interesting form of diagnosis based on the electrical conductance of acupuncture points. It was known as Electro-Acupuncture according to Voll (now known as Electro Dermal Screening). With this method, Bob was able to analyze the energetics of my body, gaining insight into the functional capacity of my organs, and determine the likely causes of stress on my system. Bob told me that a major source of stress on my body was from mercury. I had heard before of the potential for people to become ill from mercury in their fillings. I subsequently had my mercury fillings removed by Howard Hindin, DDS, and immediately felt some improvement energetically. As it turns out, this was all the beginning of what became an odyssey of many years.

I subsequently worked with health practitioners in many different fields, all the while improving my health and developing an understanding of the role of interdisciplinary healthcare.

Over the years, I continued my study and training, seeking to advance my skills in dentistry and keep up with advances in dental technology as well as broaden and deepen my understanding of the interrelationships between the mouth and the rest of the body. This book, *The Dental Connection*™, which I conceived initially in the early 1980s, is a product of that journey.

CHAPTER I
Anti-aging Dentistry?

As we get older, our bodies change. It seems pretty natural, yet for many of us the changes that occur are not actually aging but the gradual onset of disease.

Things sneak up on us, or so it seems. We might put on a little weight. We seem to tolerate stress less easily. Our blood pressure may become more elevated. We experience more fatigue and tension in our body. Our teeth may wear, discolor, or maybe we have lost some or all of them.

As we move forward dealing with the challenges of an aging population with many in declining health, there is value in reflecting on the lessons to be learned through healing traditions from around the world. Examples would be the Chinese healing arts of acupuncture and herbal medicine and the ancient healing practices of Ayurveda from India.

There are common principles found in these and other healing practices to be applied. There is a clear health benefit to living our lives with an awareness and attunement to the natural world around us. It is health promoting to eat a diet of whole foods grown free of pesticides, antibiotics, and other contaminants. It is essential for our bodies to stay free of toxins and pollutants. It is just as important to maintain a healthy digestive and elimination system. It promotes good health to have proper posture and good habits in exercise and the rest of our bodies. Healthy self-esteem promotes the choice of healthy habits and lifestyle. These basic principles form the foundation for all holistic health practices.

In dentistry, these principles have become relevant as we have learned more about the influences of oral health on systemic health and vice versa. An anti-aging holistic approach to dental care integrates knowledge of natural healing with that of contemporary dental science and technology. A few areas of concern are discussed below.

A mouth full of old mercury fillings can contribute to heavy metal toxicity causing all kinds of effects within the body, including fatigue. Research is showing that mercury from silver fillings can contribute to the development of Alzheimer's disease. Mercury toxicity has also been implicated in other neurologic and autoimmune disorders, such as MS. It is amazing that 50% of dentists still believe it is okay to keep putting mercury in people's mouths.

Other influences can occur from the development of abnormal electrical fields that can be caused by the use of various metals in the mouth. Fortunately, with advances in technology, most dentistry can be performed virtually metal free.

Crowded, crooked teeth, and a bad bite resulting from poor development of the jaws and face can contribute to a broad range of health problems in kids and adults. This may include such problems as headache, learning disabilities, digestive problems, poor posture and scoliosis, and improper breathing and constrictions of the airway leading to snoring and sleep apnea, which can impact both heart and brain health.

Did you know that years of treating your mouth one tooth at time can lead to a situation where the teeth barely look and fit like your teeth did when you were younger? This can result in worn teeth or crowns that are flat and misshapen. Often a consequence is that the bite may be uneven causing all kinds of stress throughout the body, including head, neck, and back pain, as well as other ailments.

My practice treated a woman who suffered from anxiety and from an irregular heartbeat. This was a major disruption for her, causing her to travel throughout the country seeking a solution. She found her way to our office, and we discovered that an imbalance of her bite was disrupting muscles in her neck and chest, leading to heart rhythm abnormalities. Her problem was resolved by the correct dental treatment to fix her bite and bring the muscles of her jaw, neck, and chest into balance.

We also treated a gentleman who had been experiencing nausea and elevated blood pressure. This had started after some bridgework had been done on his upper front teeth. It turned out that the new bridge compounded an underlying problem of his bite, interfering with the natural movement of his skull bones as well as affecting his jaw muscles. The result was changes in the mechanisms responsible for maintaining equilibrium and regulating blood pressure. The symptoms resolved when we corrected the bite problems by balancing the forces between his bite and the moveable bones within the skull that will be discussed in chapter V.

Research into the relationships between periodontal disease and systemic illness provides a deeper understanding of the nature of disease in general, as well as the associations between systemic and oral health. Bleeding gums and that film that coats your teeth are caused by dental plaque that can affect your heart and your major blood vessels, cause an increased risk of stroke, influence diabetes, and has been associated with pancreatic and prostate cancer as well as other health conditions. Inflammation is a common denominator between gum disease and systemic disorders.

There are various factors that may generate inflammation in your body overall, and when present, they will promote more inflammation in your gums. These systemic issues are caused by nutritional deficiencies, toxicity, faulty digestion, and stresses on the immune system from eating foods you are sensitive to.

Based on principles of natural healing, the methods of a holistic approach will help identify if there are hidden or unidentified sources of dental stress in your mouth that may contribute to the process of aging or the development of disease in your body.

The following is a list of dental conditions that may impact your health. These are considered dental risk factors that affect your general health and overall sense of well-being.

- Allergy or toxicity related to dental materials

- Infection and inflammation of the gums

- Decaying teeth leading to infections

- Teeth with failing root canals

- Residual bone cavitations in the jaw

- Electromagnetic currents created by electro-galvanic dental metals

- Imbalance of the bite or misalignment of the jaws causing neurologic, neuromuscular, cranial sacral, and myofascial tension

- Restrictions of the airway leading to snoring or sleep apnea (as well as dental stress caused by malocclusion preventing deep restorative sleep)

- Discoloration or disfigurement of the teeth affecting your self-image and comfort in smiling

In the pages that follow, I will discuss these risk factors in greater depth so you might gain more insight into those that may be impacting your health or that of a loved one. You will also develop an understanding of the benefits of a holistic approach to dentistry that cares for the health of your teeth and your mouth with your overall well-being in mind.

CHAPTER II

An Introduction to the Holistic Philosophy

"The doctor [dentist] of the future will give no medication, but
will interest his patients in the care of the human frame, diet,
and in the cause and prevention of disease."
—Thomas Edison

Introduction to the Holistic Philosophy

We have sought to understand our biological nature through the examination and dissection of ourselves and the world around us, hoping to find through an understanding of our parts that which would make us whole. This has led us to a fragmented view. With all the knowledge we have of our parts and how they work, we have not come to understand our essence.

Our view has been to see ourselves as distinct entities—similar, but separate from one another and the world around us. Because of this sense of separateness, we have evolved to see ourselves as outside of nature rather than as an expression of nature.

In the philosophy of eastern cultures, there has been a perspective that all things of the universe exist as expressions of an innate intelligence that exists as a field of energy. The intelligence within localized areas of this energy field gives expression on the planes of matter to chemical and physical entities, as well as life itself. This is now validated by the evolving fields of quantum physics and quantum biology.

Health is the result of the maintenance of an ordered state of our physiology over time. Our organism is highly evolved to adapt to changes in various environmental conditions. The more extreme these conditions are, the more adaptation we need to make and the more our physiology is stressed. With sustained stress, our systems expend their adaptive capacities, and organization of the system decays. Health is the ability of our system to maintain a highly organized state of function, what scientists call homeostasis.

Loss of health occurs because of an organism's less than optimal state of function as a whole or because of deterioration of the systems functional components. This dysfunction leads to a serial decay of the integrity of the organism as a whole resulting in disease. This process is commonly associated with the aging process, though it is truly not aging. There is abundant evidence that human beings can maintain a highly functioning state of health throughout their lifespan, though this is a relatively uncommon experience.

This deterioration of the integrity of the system, the loss of order, and the deterioration of function leads to disruptions of the body—energetically, biochemically, structurally, and functionally—ultimately creating the conditions we call disease.

Study of the world's great traditions of natural healing reveals certain truths that can be applied to promote health and well-being. Amongst these are the need for healthful nourishment, the elimination of toxins, and the maintenance of physical, emotional, and energetic balance. These basic principles form the foundation for all holistic health practices.

When disease is present, it may be viewed as evidence of a disruption in the life force. Rather than just treating the consequences of disease, a holistic practitioner is oriented to finding the cause and where possible, assisting the affected individual in reversing the disease process.

Often the cause is traced to an individual's lifestyle, their diet, their environment, their attitudes and beliefs, etc. Once the causative factors are known and eliminated, the patient's natural healing forces will resolve the "dis-ease." Healing occurs from within the individual. It cannot be imposed upon them.

Holistic Integrative Medicine is an emerging paradigm for healthcare that integrates principles of healing and health promotion from the art and science of different health professions in different cultures. The unity of the human being in mind, body, and spirit is central to the philosophy and principles employed.

For dentistry, this model is exemplified by the recognition of the mouth as a holographic microenvironment of the body and as an integral part of a whole. The art and science of dentistry have evolved in far-reaching ways since the days of our ancestors. Despite our technological advances, we still have not come to a complete and integrated understanding of the interrelationships between the mouth and the sum total of our being. There is much to learn on this subject from advances being made in many different fields of study.

In many respects, we seek truth with blinders on. We have been prejudiced by history and our personal past experience. The historical events that have guided the evolution of the dental profession have shaped our thinking and molded our beliefs about dental health and dental healthcare.

In a bygone era, a dental practitioner's scope was limited to the filling of cavities with crude materials, extracting infected teeth, and replacing them with primitive prosthetic devices. The materials used were often toxic, and the dentures sometimes created stress on the patient due to poor fit and design.

Today, the scope of dental practice has broadened immensely to encompass a wide range of sophisticated services. In essence, dentistry has progressed from concerns about only teeth to concerns about teeth, gums, and the preservation of teeth with diseased nerves (which is not always a good idea, as we will discuss later on). With the coming of age of implant dentistry, we have developed sophisticated means to replace lost teeth.

Over the past thirty years, the dental profession has become more knowledgeable in understanding the relationship between the bite and the function of the jaw joint and muscles of the head and neck.

In recent years, many advances in research have begun to reveal associations between periodontal disease and chronic systemic diseases such as cardiovascular disease, diabetes, and cancer. One could say that if this trend continues, we might just discover there is a body attached.

All along we have looked at the mouth from the perspective of dentistry, as well we should. However, as Einstein taught us with his theory of relativity, the perspective of an observer influences what she or he will see. Therefore, it is time we take a broader perspective.

A Historical Perspective: How Did We Get Here?

In the traditions of natural healing that originated in India, known as Ayurveda, healing is described as the process of the body remembering its identity. That is, to remember its "self." This is profound.

When we look at the process of disease evolving in our bodies, we may recognize that disease is the result of the body moving away from its self. Where initially there was order and organization, over time chaos ensues. This becomes expressed in the most extreme of diseases such as cancer where cells of the body cease to recognize they are part of a whole and take on an identity of their own.

A fundamental principle of Ayurvedic medicine is to re-establish the balance of mind/body/spirit through balancing the chakras. Chakras are energetic centers of the body that align with the energy or life force. Each of the seven different chakras is associated with various ailments and areas of the body. More will be discussed about chakras in chapter X, "The Body, Mind, and Mouth as Thought and Emotion."

A deeper understanding of our nature and our place in the universe can also be found in an exploration of the paradigm presented by Chinese medicine. From its conception, Chinese medicine dealt with the relationship between man and the cosmos in which we live. The energy of the universe is Chi. Chi is the energy of life. Chi exists in a myriad of forms. Practitioners of the Chinese healing arts have understood this for thousands of years.

It wasn't until Albert Einstein gave birth to quantum physics and his formula "$E = mc^2$" that the western world began to awaken to appreciate the energy within nature. We now understand that there is both a continuum and a sameness between energy and matter. As we explore this continuum, we shall appreciate the continuity and sameness between biological energy, biological chemistry, and biological structures. This will give us a foundation for understanding in more depth the Dental Connection™.

Where Did Western Medicine Get Off Track?

Concepts of natural healing have evolved in all parts of the world and in many cultures. How is it that today there seems to be such a gap between medicine as practiced in the west and what we are relearning about traditions of natural healing from around the world? How have we forgotten so much? There are probably a variety of influences.

Some relate this to the evolution of the process of scientific inquiry that evolved in the west from Descartes and Newton, etc., leading to a reductionistic manner of investigation where the whole was viewed as merely the sum of its parts. Dissect the whole and study its parts, understand them, and you understand the whole. That was the reasoning anyway.

The evolution of western scientific philosophy and technology has brought us into the modern world where our life span has improved because we don't succumb to infectious disease and malnutrition, which still affects so many in the third world countries, yet we live long enough to suffer the ravages of chronic degenerative disease. Where has modern medicine gone wrong?

Another major influence in the United States occurred shortly after the turn of the last century. In the late 1800s, there was a strong interest and widespread practice of principles of natural healing, some evolving here in the U.S. and others being imported from the natural healing traditions of Europe.

The chiropractic profession and the osteopathic profession were gaining wide support because of their effectiveness in providing relief to many who suffered from physical pain and disability. They both originated in America's Midwest. Concepts of natural healing through fasting and the use of herbal medicines were brought from Europe by Benedict Lust who founded the American School of Naturopathy.

This emergence of a natural health movement in the United States was profoundly impeded by the publication of The Flexner Report in 1910. An educator, Abraham Flexner was commissioned by Andrew Carnegie to study the quality of medical education in the United States and make recommendations for its improvement. His report, which was broad in its scope of recommendations, led to many improvements in the quality of training of allopathic physicians (MDs). Unfortunately, there were negative consequences as well.

"When Flexner developed his report, allopathic medicine faced vigorous competition from several quarters, including osteopathic medicine, naturopathic medicine, eclectic medicine, physio-medicine, herbal medicine and homeopathic medicine."[1]

Flexner had a firm conviction that the physician should be scientific

---

1. 'Flexner Report', *Wikipedia* http://en.wikipedia.org/wiki/Flexner_Report.

in his approach to treat disease. In his time, the only field of science that had firmly established itself was the field of chemistry; the fields of biology and physics were in relative infancy.

In the field of medicine, the discipline of surgery was well established. Much advance had been made on the battlefields of the Civil War and in the subsequent years.

There had been much success preventing and treating infectious disease following the emergence of the germ theory in the late 1800s and applying the ideas of antisepsis introduced to the hospital setting by Joseph Lister. Lister had introduced the use of carbolic acid (now known as phenol) applied to surgical dressings to prevent infection as well as the concept of sterilization of surgical instruments.

Physicians had also been using chemical compounds to alter the physiological effects associated with disease. Aspirin had been introduced by the Bayer Company of Germany for the treatment of pain in 1899. It was the first non-addictive pain medication.

In 1903, barbiturates were introduced as a sedative, and were soon to replace the use of bromides that had been used to relieve symptoms of headache and stress. (Bromides were used in products such as Bromo-seltzer and were found eventually to be toxic and discontinued in use following WWII.)

Flexner, therefore, declared that to be scientific the physician needed to restrict his treatments to the use of chemical or surgical interventions. Flexner believed that any form of medicine other than allopathy that didn't employ drug therapies to treat disease was the same as quackery and charlatanism.

"Medical schools that offered courses in bioelectric medicine, eclectic medicine, naturopathy, homeopathy, or 'eastern medicine', for example, were told either to drop these courses from their curriculum or lose their accreditation and underwriting support. A few schools resisted for a time, but eventually all complied with the Flexner Report or shut their doors. This led to the standardization of the curricula of surviving schools."[2]

It is of interest to note that in 1930 Flexner cofounded the **Institute for Advanced Study**, located in Princeton, New Jersey. Albert Einstein was one of the first professors that Flexner recruited there.[3] By this point, Flexner recognized that science was broader than what the field of chemistry alone had considered.

But the die was cast, and the evolution of medicine and dentistry (which sought to follow the "scientific model" of medical education) continued for almost one hundred years following an allopathic model seeking to counter disease states of the body with surgery and chemical formulas, but gaining little more understanding of the nature of chronic degenerative disease.

2. 'Flexner Report', *Wikipedia* https://en.wikipedia.org/wiki/Flexner_Report.
3. 'Albert Einstein', *Historical Society of Princeton*, https://princetonhistory.org/research/historic-princeton/albert-einstein/.

CHAPTER III
Our Energy Body and the Mouth

A s we embrace knowledge drawn from ancient concepts of healing such as Ayurveda and Chinese medicine, we understand that the body is an energy field with physical form.

Chinese medicine, the medicine of energy, speaks of this energy as Qi (also known as Chi). Chi is the energy of life. Chi exists in a myriad of forms. The Chinese have understood this for thousands of years. It wasn't until Albert Einstein gave birth to quantum physics and his formula $E = mc^2$ that the western world began to awaken to this. We now understand that there is a continuum and sameness between energy and matter. All is one. Sound familiar? We are an expression of nature and the field of the universe. We maintain health to the degree we maintain the order of our being in harmony with those conditions that promote life.

These ancient concepts have now been explained by the concepts of modern science such as quantum physics and the related field of biophysics. These concepts are well described in the book *Energy Medicine: The Scientific Basis* by James Oschman, and explored further on his website.[4] This book is a must-read for anyone wanting a more in-depth understanding of the energetic nature of biologic systems.

The energy pathways of the body, known in Chinese medicine as the meridians, run from our feet through our torso, neck, and head, along our arms to our fingertips and back down again to our feet. As they pass through the body, they follow along pathways that course through the skin and underlying fascia, our muscles and bones, through our organs, and through the skull and teeth. Every cell of the body is in communication with every other cell via this connective tissue energy internet.

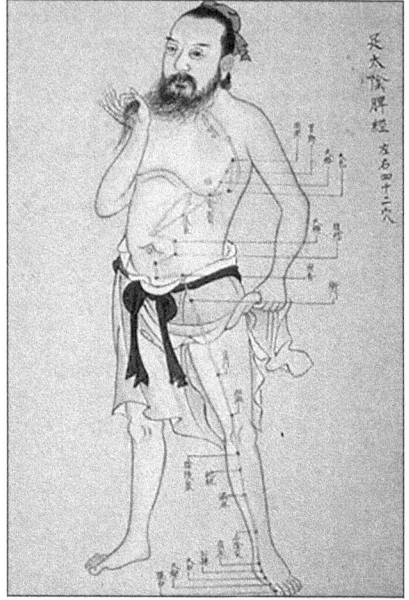

Figure 1: The Liver Meridian from an ancient drawing

The terms Yang and Yin used in the Chinese model of acupuncture energetics reflect the duality of Qi as seen in nature and the balancing push/pull of energy. This manifests as day and night, light and dark, hot and cold, up and down, male and female, etc. Interestingly, again there are parallels in contemporary western thought introduced by Einstein's Theory of Relativity. In our bodies, we can think of Yin as energy that flows into our body from outside and Yang energy that flows from our bodies to the external environment. A general rule is that "Yang will tend to excess, and Yin will tend toward deficiency."

The simple act of walking in nature drives an energy exchange that can be healing. There is an energy exchange between the earth and the body with every step. A bare foot enhances the transfer and provides

---

4. 'James L. Oschman', *Energy Medicine University*, http://www.energymedicineuniversity. org/
faculty/oschman.html.

natural changes to the energy state. All meridians of the body pass through the ball of the foot and absorb the positive energy of the earth. This creates the effect called "grounding."

In the West, we speak of circulation systems in the body pertaining to the flow of fluids, primarily blood and lymph. In Chinese medicine, a broader view is taken with the flow of fluids being only a component of the overall flow of energy through the body's tissues.

Chinese medicine views the flow of energy as occurring through a network of channels, known as meridians, both on the surface and deep within the body. Access to influence the flow of energy through the body is afforded by the presence of acupuncture points that manifest along meridians on the surface.

Energetic therapies like acupuncture provide patients with the release of chronic tension and pain caused by previous traumas and other adverse effects of the body. Acupuncture gives comfort to individuals by bringing them closer to their true selves, facilitating the body's energy flow. In this way, the client's body is freed of discomfort and debilitating conditions.[5] Similar results can be achieved through other forms of therapy that deal with the continuity of the body's tissues such as cranial sacral therapy, osteopathy, and chiropractic. All of these methods assist the body in restoring "homeostasis."

Stimulation of points along these meridians will have an influence on remote, related organs and tissues. For example, "When acupuncture points on the kidney meridian are stimulated, they affect not only the kidney, but also embryologically related organs such as the ovary, testicle, uterus, fallopian tube, and to some extent the adrenal."[6]

This is because, as the information encoded in our DNA is manifesting in response to the evolving energy fields of the embryo, tissues

5. Mark Seem, *A New American Acupuncture: Acupuncture Osteopathy - The Myofascial Release of The Bodymind's Holding Patterns.* (BluePoppy Press, 1993).
6. Felix Mann, *The Ancient Chinese Art of Healing and How It Works Scientifically,* 2nd edition (Vintage Books, 1973).

differentiate and at the same time maintain energetic connections to the germ tissues of their origin. Organs and tissues originating in different germ layers and regions of the nascent embryo share connections to their embryologic roots, thus the holographic nature of the body.

The meridians develop as our embryo is formed and begins to define us. As the initial fertilization of the egg by sperm occurs and the egg then divides in two, the first meridian relationship is formed because there are now two cells with an interface between them where they now have an electromagnetic relationship.

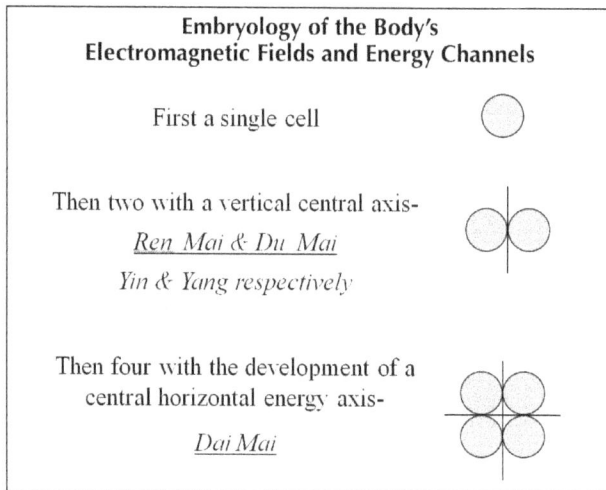

Embryology of the Body's Electromagnetic Fields and Energy Channels

First a single cell

Then two with a vertical central axis-
Ren Mai & Du Mai
Yin & Yang respectively

Then four with the development of a central horizontal energy axis-
Dai Mai

Figure 2: The author's conception of the development of the meridians

This electromagnetic relationship continues to evolve and become more complex. It is persistent throughout our growth and development, as well as during our life. The connective tissues and the energetic relationships that develop provide for the continuity and relatedness of all of the cells within our body.

The major pathways of energy flow, defined as the Regular Meridians, are twelve pathways of energy flow that manifest along the superficial tissues of the body. They run from hand to head, from head to the foot, and vice versa. These meridians are known by the names of the organs (Zang Fu) with which they are related such as Lung, Large Intestine, Stomach, Spleen, Heart, Small Intestine, Bladder, Kidney, Pericardium, Triple Warmer [not actually an organ in the western sense, it relates to the balancing of energy, most closely related to our endocrine system], and Gall Bladder.

These Regular Meridians have subsidiary branches called divergent and collateral meridians that supply areas of the body adjacent to them. The divergent meridians run interiorly, and the collateral meridians run superficially. Keep in mind that the meridians incorporate every cell of the body.

For a basic understanding, consider that the meridians that are described as Yin are related to the organs involved with energy flowing into and circulating deep within the body. They arise from the feet and course deep within the body through the torso, head, and teeth to the tips of the fingers. Therefore, we have the Kidney, Liver, and Spleen arising in the feet (around the arch of the foot and the big toe) flowing into the torso and the head, and then the Heart, Pericardium, and Lung flowing into the hands to the tips of the fingers.

The meridians described as Yang run more superficially. They run down the back of the hands through the head and teeth to the torso, back down the legs and then through the heel and lateral part of the forefoot back to the ground. Originating in the hands, these are the meridians of Small Intestine, Triple Warmer (related to the flow of energy through the torso), and Large Intestine, which flow to the head and teeth and their continuation is as Bladder, Gall Bladder, and Stomach flowing down through the body to the feet.

These twelve Regular Meridians are described in *Chinese Acupuncture and Moxibustion* as "conduits which distribute Qi (Chi) and blood of the twelve major meridians to nourish the muscles, and possess the function of connecting all the bones and joints of the body in the maintenance of the normal range of motion."[7]

---

7. Ibid.

The Teeth Are Connected to All Parts of the Body through the Meridians

The teeth are connected by the meridians to all parts of the body. The Chinese did not describe this. This fact was first described by Rheinhold Voll, M.D., in the 1950s. He invented a device known as the Dermatron with which he could measure variances in the galvanic skin response at different acupuncture points. In turn, he was able to stimulate acupuncture points that were out of balance to encourage a return to balance.

As he gained experience over time, his success in treatment continued to improve, and he made several important discoveries. One of the most important was the relationship of the teeth to the meridians. Voll discovered that when a tooth was diseased or had a toxic material used in a dental restoration, it impeded the healing of his patients. In other words, disease within the teeth will influence other regions of the body and vice versa. See Figure 3 on the next page.

This is readily demonstrated by means of Applied Kinesiology reflex testing as well as Voll electro-acupuncture diagnosis. When the teeth are diseased or stressed and acting as an influence elsewhere in the body, they are defined as being a focus of irritation within the energy systems of the body. The most common condition of a tooth that results in it acting as a focus is when the tooth has become infected because of a degenerative condition of the nerve pulpal tissue, which often results in root canal treatment of the tooth. Frequently, root canal treated teeth will act as persistent foci despite the appearance of a successful root canal treatment. More on this in Chapter VIII, "Focal Infection: a Challenge to the Immune System."

Another important part of the mouth's influence on the energetic body arises from the relationship of the bite to the function of the body as a whole. Because each tooth and the jaw system itself are connected to the body's energy internet, too much pressure from the bite on an individual tooth has the potential to short circuit its associated meridian.

This can result in weakness of muscles or stress on the organ associated with the muscle.

Misalignment of the jaw structures may also disrupt the flow through the meridians, as well as contribute to misalignment and imbalance of major structural elements of the body including the cranial sacral and musculoskeletal system. This will be discussed in more detail in Chapter V, "Our Physical Body and the Mouth."

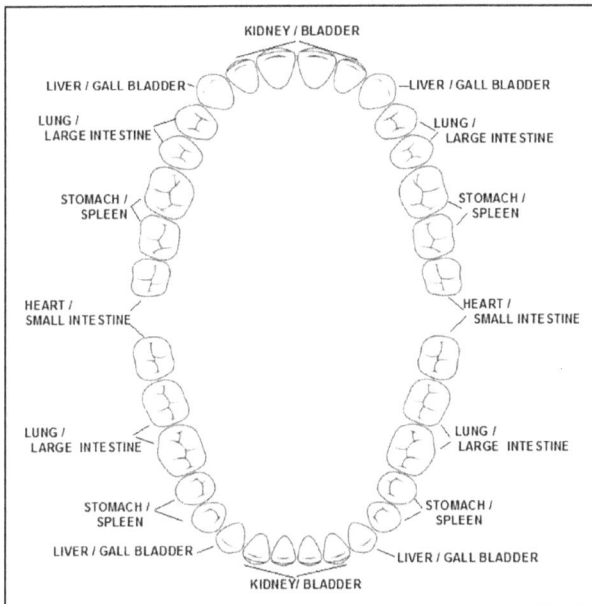

Figure 3: Voll's Dental Meridian Connections

When concerned about our general health, it is important to consider the energy connections to the mouth, jaw, and teeth. As stated, the tissues of the mouth and teeth are connected energetically to all other parts of the body. Each tooth corresponds with a different energetic pathway including the organ associated with it.

CHAPTER IV
Our Biochemical Body and the Mouth
Nutrition and Degenerative Dental Disease

"There are so many health issues that are caused or perpetuated by problems in the mouth that the dental division of a comprehensive center is indispensable."
—Dietrich Klinghardt, M.D., Ph.D.

My favorite subjects in college were the overlapping fields of biochemistry and molecular biology. I was fascinated by these subjects because they spoke about the alphabet soup of substances and processes that defined life.

Definition of some terms is in order here. To paraphrase the words of Albert Lehninger Ph.D., author of my college text of biochemistry[8], "Biochemistry is the language that describes the energetic principles that govern how living things take in energy from their environment, transform and use it, and then discharge it back into their environment." (Sounds like Yin and Yang).

Molecular biology is essentially the study of the structures and inner workings of our cells, and it explores how our biochemistry works in cell function, including the expression of our DNA. Much has been discovered in the past 100 years in these fields that give us a deeper, though still incomplete, understanding of the nature of life. These fields

---

8. Albert Lehninger, *Principles of Biochemistry* (Worth Publishers, 1970).

have somewhat melded together, giving rise to what today is called quantum (energetic) biology.

So, where does this energy of life come from? Our food, as well as the water we drink, the air we breathe, and our electromagnetic environment. This would seem to be a simple matter if all the food we ate was of equal quality. But it is not. Nor is our drinking water of equal quality.

Webster Dictionary defines food as "material consisting essentially of protein, carbohydrate, and fat used in the body of an organism to sustain growth, repair damage, to support our vital processes and to furnish energy." If it were as simple as that, it wouldn't matter what the qualities of our food were if we met our requirements for protein, carbohydrate, and fat. Quite the contrary, however, as the quality of our food does matter and profoundly impacts both our dental and systemic health, as we shall see.

While we have much in common, we are all genetically different, reflecting the biologic history of our ancestors. Wherever they originated on the globe, they evolved eating a diet probably different than we are eating today. Anthropologic study has shown that if our distant ancestors had an adequate and varied diet, they probably enjoyed good dental health. In recent generations, things have changed, and despite all our modern technology and conveniences, our access to nutritious meals has deteriorated.

From the very beginning, living things have derived their source of nutrients from their environment. Initially, the single cell organisms that arose out of the primordial soup extracted nutrients from the environment immediately outside of their membranes, as our cells still do.

As life evolved, multicellular organisms took their nutrients into their stoma (the opening directly into their stomach) from their external environment. Plants drew energy from the sun and nutrients from the soil. Animals evolved that ate the plants, and then other animals evolved that ate other animals. Eventually, Homo sapiens evolved. Our ancestors were hunter-gatherers. They ate mostly plant-based sources of foods: leaves, stalks, roots, seeds, fruits, and vegetables. They learned to hunt. When successful, they ate animal proteins.

About 10,000 years ago, our ancestors learned to cultivate grains (seeds from grasses). As agriculture continued to evolve, it supported the development of large stable communities. Fast forward to the modern era where large cities have emerged all over the globe and now most of us live far removed from farms, forests, fields, and the sea; the source of our food supply.

Most food today is produced on an industrial scale with manmade chemicals introduced to improve the yield and preserve freshness. In our supermarkets, most of the food has been processed and modified, packaged in boxes and cans or frozen. Only by conscious awareness can we shop and replicate a diet that comes close to that of our ancestors.

Our biochemistry is being disrupted due to elements and chemical compounds introduced into our systems to which our ancestors had not been exposed. Our consumption of "foods" that are not truly nourishing us is worsening the problem. Today, chronic degenerative diseases such as cardiovascular disease, cancer, arthritis, Alzheimer's, diabetes, and a host of autoimmune diseases have become a common occurrence as we age. These are all disorders involving nutrient deficiencies, chronic toxicity, and inflammation.

Back in 1910 when Flexner redirected the attention of medicine to focus on treating disease with "magic bullets," the field of chemistry had not yet become the field of biochemistry that we know today. There were many changes occurring in all of the emerging sciences. As the field of chemistry had been evolving in the late 1800s, in other arenas, scientists were using microscopes to examine the world of living things invisible to the naked eye.

The role that the "bugs" in our mouth played in the development of tooth decay and periodontal disease was discovered by W.D. Miller during the golden age of microbiology in the late 1800s. Inspired by Pasteur's research into bacteria fermenting sugars into lactic acid, and Emil Magitot studying the fermentation of sugars dissolving teeth in the laboratory, Miller developed his own oral microbiological research. He developed numerous research projects that introduced modern biological principles to dentistry.

In 1890, Miller formulated the theory that tooth decay (caries) is caused by acids produced by oral bacteria following fermentation of sugars. He described how dental caries were the result of fermentation of carbohydrates in the mouth by microorganisms[9]. His research established the foundation for our understanding of the role of microorganisms in both tooth decay and periodontal disease.

Miller also spoke about the potential for bacteria originating in the mouth to contribute to systemic disease, an idea that gained favor in the early 1900s as the Focal Infection Theory, only to be discarded as medicine was influenced by Flexner's dictum of "be scientific."[10] At the time, there was a lack of understanding of how the interactions between the mouth and body could occur.

It was not until the 1980s that it became more generally accepted that oral bacteria can contribute to cardiac disease and other potentially serious illnesses. This will be explored below in the discussion of periodontal disease as well as in Chapter VIII, "Focal Infection: Challenge to the Immune System."

In 1924, J. Kilian Clark published the paper *On the Bacterial Factor in the Etiology of Dental Caries*. In this paper, he described his discovery of a specific bacterium that produced tooth decay. He proposed the name Streptococcus mutans to describe it. He stated that this bacterium would ferment sugars producing a highly acidic environment on the surface of the tooth that would generate decay. As the field of

---

9. 'Willoughby D. Miller', *Wikipedia*, https://en.wikipedia.org/wiki/Willoughby_D._Miller.
10. Ibid.

microbiology was developing, so too was the field of biochemistry and the understanding of the role of nutrition in the development of both dental and systemic disease.

One of the most prominent researchers in the field of nutrition who contributed greatly to our understanding of the role of nutrition in human health was Weston Price, DDS. He was a respected dental researcher and amateur anthropologist who published a classic work in 1939 titled, *Nutrition and Physical Degeneration - A Comparison of Primitive and Modern Diets and Their Effects.*[11]

He found that in societies living in isolation from the modern world and eating traditional native diets, the occurrence of degenerative dental disease was uncommon. His findings were based on observations of people living in isolated communities that until recently had not been exposed to modern foods. People living all over the globe in different climates were observed, including the Loteshental in the Swiss Alps, Native Americans, Polynesians, Pygmies, and Aborigines.

Those who held to the dietary traditions of their ancestors thrived. Those who deviated developed signs of physical degeneration. Introduction of modern processed foods such as sugar, white flour, and processed vegetable fats led to degenerative changes in the body chemistry leading to rampant tooth decay and maldevelopment of orofacial structures.

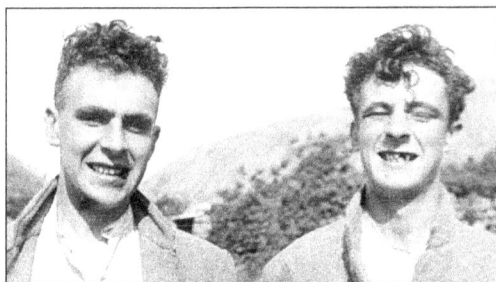

Figure 4: Two Gaelic brothers eating different diets
© Price-Pottenger Nutrition Foundation, Inc.
All rights reserved. www.ppnf.org

In this photo of two Gaelic brothers, we can see the brother on the left with a broad face and healthy smile who had eaten a native diet.

The brother on the right has a narrowed, less symmetrical face, and has developed

11. Weston Price, *Nutrition and Physical Degeneration: A Comparison of Primitive and Modern Diets and Their Effects* (Keats Pub., 1990).

rampant tooth decay. His diet was mostly white flour, sugar, and other modern foods.

The degeneration manifested itself as tooth decay and gum disease in adults eating the processed foods. Now we understand more about the role of nutrition in chronic degenerative disease.

In children, mal-development of the orofacial structures became apparent. These problems that developed with children were due to direct and indirect consequences of malnutrition. Due to the insult to the immune system in their gut, these children would likely have developed allergies leading to airway disorders that contributed to the development of bite disorders, as well as other health problems.

Dr. Price's findings were supported by thousands of photographs showing the impact after the introduction of de-natured foods. Some of these photos are reproduced here.

In these photos, we see examples of normal and proper development of orofacial structures in both the two native American girls as well as the two adult males from the Belgian Congo.

Figure 5: People eating healthy diets

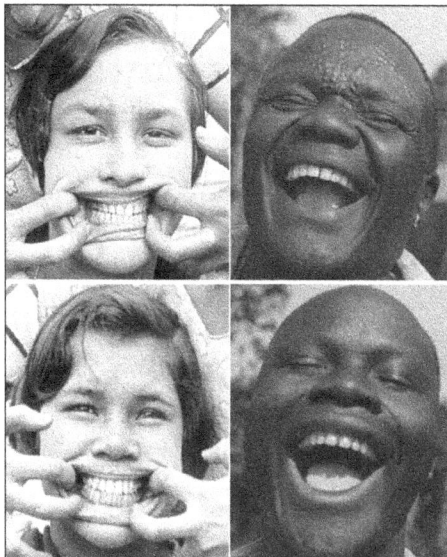

In these photos, we see examples of degenerative changes with people consuming western foods. The two children with developing mal-occlusion were native to northern Canada. The two adults were living in Africa and had rampant tooth decay.

**Figure 6: The dental consequences of
eating Western processed foods**

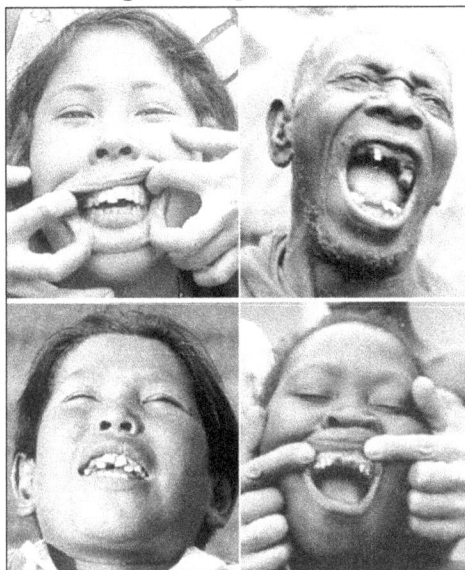

Another giant in the field of nutrition and dental disease was Harold F. Hawkins, DDS. He published *Applied Nutrition*[12] in 1947, writing about his research into the role of nutrition in the development of dental decay and gum disease. He demonstrated that the imbalances of body chemistry associated with chronic degenerative dental diseases such as tooth decay and periodontal disease could be restored to a balanced equilibrium that promoted health through a program of dietary modification and the judicious use of vitamins and supplements.

His research spanned the course of twenty years, studying over eight thousand cases. His research was directed to understanding why

---

12. Harold F Hawkins, D.D.S., *Applied Nutrition* (Mojave Books, 1947).

some were prone to decay and others had relative immunity.

He reasoned that since the process of decay was a biochemical one, perhaps the factors that conveyed immunity against decay could be understood by studying the variability of oral biochemistry. He found those immune to decay maintained an effective means of neutralizing the acidity caused by the fermentation of carbohydrates in the mouth. This occurs through several different mechanisms.

1) The effect of the acids generated could be neutralized by the buffering capacity of:

   a. soluble alkaline salts of potassium, sodium, and magnesium

   b. insoluble salts of calcium in fine suspension or in a colloidal state

   c. the presence of mucin, a glycoprotein secreted by salivary glands which creates the mucoid quality of saliva

2) The concentration and therefore the effect of the acids could be reduced by dilution.

Sufficient dilution of an acid reduces its ability to act chemically on calcium salts.

Hawkins found that 74% of those who were decay prone had a deficiency in the amount of saliva, whereas only 23% of those immune to decay did. Most dentists today would agree based on their clinical experience that dryness of the mouth contributes to tooth decay.

The saliva of the "decay immune" has sufficient neutralizing capacity to reduce the effects of the acid and afford protection to the teeth. Those prone to decay do not. The volume and quality of the saliva is an important protective factor as well.

Further investigation allowed Hawkins to demonstrate why a diet high in carbohydrates yielded an increase in tooth decay. He demonstrated that another important variable was the level of salivary amylase, a digestive enzyme secreted in saliva that acts upon starches in the mouth. His study showed that 66% of those who were decay prone were deficient in amylase whereas only 24% of those immune to decay had equally low levels.

The level of amylase was found related to two factors:

1) The amount of vitamin B in the diet, which influences amylase production

2) The amount of carbohydrates or sugars in the diet. Carbohydrates and sugars consume the amylase as it breaks them down.

If these factors are out of balance or below normal, they will have to be corrected in order for decay to be controlled or prevented. It may call for a change in the level of the minerals, vitamins, and digestive and endocrine secretions, as well as a change in the dietary habits of the patient.

Hawkins recognized that the white flour and processed starches and sugars in the diet of these individuals had been processed to remove the nutrient rich bran from the grain, which is high in B vitamins. Our bodies need these B vitamins to manufacture amylase.

A student of Hawkins, John E. Waters, DDS, observed associations between heavy tartar formation and difficulty with fat assimilation that would be responsive to treatment with bile salts. After a period of a few months consuming supplemental bile salts, the problems of tartar accumulation would disappear.

He observed an association between this excessive tartar buildup and the eventual onset of serious diseases like cancer when left untreated. He published his findings in the article "Correctable Systemic Disorders Indicated by Presence of Salivary Calculus." He believed that chronic periodontitis was a systemic disease. "Local treatment but reduces the obvious symptoms; it does not affect the basic disease."[13]

His observations were made during the years he served on the staff of a county hospital where patients were grouped into wards according to their medical conditions. In the surgical ward with a high proportion of accident cases, he observed that most patients did not have heavy tartar. In wards with chronically ill patients, every patient had calculus, and it was usually heavy. Of these, many wore dentures also with heavy tartar deposits.

Waters discussed his observations with his mentor Dr. Hawkins, and they arrived at the following conclusion: "There appears to be in certain fats a factor. They called it factor F for simplicity. F factor controls the selective function of the kidneys in selecting from the bloodstream the acid wastes of life's processes and eliminating them via the urine. When factor F is not adequate in the diet, the acid waste is not eliminated properly. It remains in the bloodstream, to result in a systemic acidosis. In turn, the saliva being made from that more-than-normally-acidic blood precipitates solids on the teeth in the form known as dental calculus."[14]

The presence of heavy salivary calculus buildup on the teeth was discovered to be a component of impaired immune system efficiency and metabolism.

By studying chronically ill patients and confirming the dental connection, Waters justified his hypothesis that health issues can be improved when the biochemical imbalance that underlies the formation of salivary calculus on the teeth is corrected.

Melvin Page, DDS, was another great in the field of clinical nutrition and its role in dental health. He looked at the work of Weston Price and took it a step further. Like Hawkins, he looked at the biochemistry

---

13. John E. Waters, 'Correctable Systemic Disorders Indicated by Presence of Salivary Calculus', *Selene River Press*, https://www.seleneriverpress.com/historical/correctable-systemic-disorders-indicated-by-presence-of-salivary-calculus/.
14. Ibid.

involved but focused on changes in the blood chemistry instead of saliva. In thousands of blood tests, Dr. Page discovered that tooth decay would stay in check when there was a precise ratio maintained between calcium and phosphorus in the blood. This ratio was 10:4.

"Dr. Page believed that body chemistry, when properly balanced by proper nutrition and other factors, will not only prevent dental problems but will naturally affect the rest of the body as well. He bluntly stated that you cannot affect the teeth through body chemistry and nutrition without having beneficial effects on the entire body."

He promoted several forward thinking ideas that met with resistance such as:

- The harmful effects of the use of sugar.

- The harmful effects of using chemical additives and other food preservatives for the sake of "shelf life."

- Using vitamins, minerals and digestive enzymes to supplement daily food intake.

- That milk is not the perfect food for everyone.

- That a person's endocrine system must be in balance for optimum physical and mental health and could be maintained through the use of micro-doses of endocrines (where warranted)."[15]

Royal Lee, DDS, believed that common practices used in food processing destroyed the nutritional quality of our food. "The chemical and thermal mauling of the food supply is precisely at the root of our ill health," he wrote in his 1961 manifesto of holistic nutrition.[16]

Dr. Lee explained that it was shortsighted to view foods solely in terms of calories, the measures of how much fuel a food supplies. He

---

15. http://www.rubysemporium.org/health/body/body-chem.html.
16. Royal Lee, *Natural Food and Farming*, 1961.

stated that processing and refining of foods does not tend to alter the caloric content of foods, but results in uncontrolled damage to the foods' non-caloric elements: the vitamins, minerals, and countless other known and unknown cofactors that spur the thousands of bio-chemical reactions required to repair and sustain the body. So while these products give the illusion of sustenance, they fail to provide the most basic level of nutrients necessary to sustain human health.

Dr. Lee subsequently developed a company called Standard Process for the production of concentrated nutrients to supplement a deficient diet and help correct health conditions caused by poor nutrition.

What Then Are the Implications for People Who Suffer from Tooth Decay or Gum Disease?

When an individual is affected with tooth decay or gum disease, con-sideration should be given to potential contributory imbalances in the chemistry of the body. One should evaluate the general balance of the biochemistry with particular attention to the pH of saliva and the levels of calcium and phosphorous in the blood. The amount and frequency of refined carbohydrate intake are also an important consideration. The overall energy state of the individual should be considered, and if defec-tive, the imbalance may be treated through modification of the diet and the use of whole food supplements to compensate for deficiencies.

Changes in the body's biochemistry will lead to conditions that favor disease. These changes that lead to disruption of the biochemical pathways are involved in repair and regeneration of body tissues. These changes can favor the growth of some types of microorganisms over others.

Tooth decay and gum disease are commonly thought to be caused by dental plaque, or growths of bacteria on the teeth. Today we are now calling this biofilm. We are recognizing that this biofilm is a highly organized community of bacteria that develops on the surface of a tooth and is influenced by the overall microbiome of the body.

Exploring how our diet impacts our microbiome provides a further understanding of the interconnectedness of our mouth, digestive system, and whole body. We now know that our health is dependent on a proper balance of the microorganisms that live within us, especially in our gut. This balance can be readily disturbed by an unhealthy diet as well as the use of drugs such as antibiotics.

We are just beginning to appreciate the relationship between "the bugs in our mouth and the bugs in our gut."

> The **microbiome** is **defined** as the collective genomes of the microbes (composed of bacteria, bacteriophage, fungi, protozoa and viruses) that live inside and on the **human** body. We have about ten times as many microbial cells as **human cells.**

Tooth Decay

As we have discussed, tooth decay is the result of a breakdown of the structure of a tooth because of acids produced by specific types of bacteria. The mineral content of the tooth is dissolved by lactic acid produced by the fermentation of sugars such as sucrose, fructose, and glucose by the bacteria Streptococcus mutans and Lactobacillus.

The mineral component of the teeth is in a state of equilibrium that remains stable as long as the pH on the surface of the tooth remains above 5.5, with a pH of 7 being optimal. In a state of health, this is readily achieved through the buffering action of saliva, which has calcium and phosphorus present in the solution.

There are many variables, unique to each individual. The role of bacteria in tooth decay and biological infirmities depends on the type of bacteria, host resistance, and the type of proteins in the saliva.

The chemistry of saliva is complex and the subject of much research today. Sialin aids the buffering capacity of saliva by countering the effects of acid production by bacteria, as does sodium bicarbonate, amphoteric proteins, and urea, which is broken down by bacteria into ammonia.[17] Statherin, a phospho-protein, acts to stabilize both calcium and phosphorus in the supersaturated saliva. This supersaturated saliva aids in preventing overall decay and improving oral wellness. This was demonstrated by the work of Weston Price.

Good oral hygiene is stressed for prevention and is essential to keep the growth of bacterial biofilms in check. A diet low in fermentable sugars as described above will reduce the risk of tooth decay. It is important as well that grains, especially processed grains, be kept to a minimum for patients at risk of tooth decay. Processed grains, in particular, may contribute to B vitamin deficiencies as well as impact the intestinal absorption of calcium.

In a "traditional" approach to dental care, fluoride is used to harden enamel to make it more resistant to decay. There have been concerns raised that this may not be as good as first thought because it is absorbed in other tissues of the body, and there are reports associating use of fluoride with higher risk of cancer. It is more sound and better for our health overall to follow a proper diet and exercise nutritional discipline, avoiding the temptations of eating sweets and other processed nutritionally deficient foods.

Periodontal Disease

Today, mainstream medicine and dentistry are awakening to The Dental Connection™ thanks to the research that has been conducted over the past few years, showing the association between gum disease and systemic

---

17. Llena-Puy, C., The role of saliva in maintaining oral health and as an aid to diagnosis. Med Oral Patol Oral Cir Bucal 2006;11:E449-55. https://pdfs.semanticscholar. org/6169/e19d6d569e3e3ca8d352cb6d65d80eab3e1f.pdf.

inflammation. While inflammation in the body has been recognized as a serious problem by functionally oriented practitioners for a long time, it is now getting to be big news because mainstream researchers are identifying the role of inflammation in many chronic, degenerative conditions.

Inflammation is not a synonym for infection. Even in cases where inflammation is caused by infection, it is incorrect to use the terms as synonyms: infection is caused by an exogenous pathogen, while inflammation is the response of the organism to the pathogen or some other irritant.

"Inflammation (Latin, inflammatio, to set on fire) is the complex biological response of vascular tissues to harmful stimuli, such as pathogens, damaged cells, or irritants. It is a protective attempt by the organism to remove the injurious stimuli as well as initiate the healing process for the tissue.

—From Wikipedia, the free encyclopedia

In the absence of inflammation, wounds and infections would never heal and progressive destruction of the tissue would compromise the survival of the organism. However, inflammation which runs unchecked can also lead to a host of diseases, such as hay fever, atherosclerosis, and rheumatoid arthritis. It is for this reason that inflammation is normally tightly regulated by the body.

Inflammation can be classified as either <u>acute</u> or <u>chronic</u>. **Acute** inflammation is the initial response of the body to harmful stimuli and is achieved by the increased movement of plasma and leukocytes from the blood into the injured tissues. A cascade of biochemical events propagates and matures the inflammatory response, involving the local vascular system, the immune system, and various cells within the injured tissue.

Prolonged inflammation, known as chronic inflammation, leads to a progressive shift in the type of cells which are present at the site of inflammation and is characterized by simultaneous destruction and healing of the tissue from the inflammatory process.[18] This is what occurs in periodontal disease.

A couple of years ago, I did a series of radio interviews with a friend who had a health-centered radio show, Dr. Rick Huntoon. We did a show on periodontal disease and the systemic links found with it. The transcript is reproduced below, and it serves as a summary of the link between periodontal disease and the body.

"I read about the links between the health of the mouth and overall systemic health, especially the associations between gum disease and health throughout the body. Tell us about gum disease."

Gum diseases, called "periodontal diseases" by dentists and physicians, are complex chronic infectious and inflammatory conditions of the gums and other tissues supporting the teeth. They may result in the destruction of tissues supporting the teeth, resulting in eventual tooth loss. As this occurs, there are systemic interactions resulting from both the generation of inflammation as well as the invasion of bacteria into the blood system as the protective barriers provided by healthy gum tissue break down.

As is the case with most disease, genetics as well as the nutritional and lifestyle habits of the individual play a major role in determining who gets gum disease, and what the consequences will be for them.

"How might someone know they have gum disease?"

Do your gums bleed? Are they red or puffy? Are any of your teeth loose? Do you think you have bad breath? Have you been told by your dentist that you need to brush better or see the hygienist more frequently? If your answer to any of these questions is yes, then you probably have some form of periodontal or gum disease.

---

18. 'Inflammation', *Wikipedia*, https://en.wikipedia.org/wiki/Inflammation.

"What is actually taking place when someone has gum disease?"

The teeth are held in the jawbones by soft tissue that is a continuation of the gum. This tissue forms a ligament, which acts as a shock absorber for the tooth. In a healthy state, this gum tissue forms a tight collar around the tooth with a space of about 1 or 2 mm above where it is attached to the tooth.

Bacteria that collect on the surface of the tooth form a sticky substance that allows more bacteria to build up. As they accumulate on the surface of the tooth, they release waste products that are toxic and irritating to the gum. Our bodies' defensive mechanisms kick in in reaction to these irritants resulting in inflammation along the edge of the gum.

When the patient is well nourished and has good host resistance, the condition stops here and the bacteria are held in check.

"What happens if the condition progresses?"

When conditions are less favorable, numerous things may happen that lead to a progression of the disease and a myriad of consequences.

As the bacteria invade the tissues, the body mounts a defensive reaction known as inflammation. We are all familiar with inflammation. Anytime we experience swelling, redness around a bruise or cut, fever, and pain, inflammation is involved. As the inflammation persists, tissues get broken down as a consequence of chemicals released by our body as well as the bacteria. We begin to lose the integrity of the tissues designed to protect the support for our teeth.

"What happens then?"

In general, as the inflammation persists and our gum tissues lose their ability to maintain a barrier, the bacteria penetrate the tissues. The inflammation (our body's response) and the infection penetrate deeper until the bone around the tooth itself begins to be affected by the inflammation and ultimately the infection. Our tissues break down, and the bone begins to decay.

"What are the consequences if gum disease is left untreated?"

Ultimately, the patient develops deep pockets around their teeth, and the gums may recede as bone continues to break down. Eventually, teeth may become loose and ultimately fall out. As bad as this is, we now understand more about the systemic effects of this ongoing chronic infection and inflammation.

"What do you mean?"

We have always thought of gum disease as a localized problem in the mouth. We now understand that its consequences are more profound than that. The bacteria associated with gum disease are known to be invasive, ultimately entering the blood stream and infecting other tissues and organs. Also, the inflammation triggered by the body's response to the gum infection will trigger and contribute to inflammation throughout the body.

"That sounds bad. Could you please tell us more about that?"

Okay, there are three parts to this.

The first is the bacteria causing the gum disease. The second part is the body's response or inflammation. The third is caused by free radicals and oxidative stress that impact the health of the tissues.

Let's start with the first part, the bacteria causing the gum disease, these bugs that grow on the surfaces of our teeth. We now know that these bugs get into our bloodstream when the protective barrier provided by healthy gum tissue is compromised by chronic gum disease and inflammation.

One of these bugs, known as S. Sanguinis, is a common part of dental plaque and has been shown to be the major cause of infected heart valves, also called infective endocarditis.

Studies have shown that the thickening of blood vessels, like the carotid artery, which supplies blood to the head and brain, is associated with the accumulation of bacteria originating in the mouth. One of the complications that can occur during pregnancy is preeclampsia. This is characterized by a sudden rise in blood pressure that occurs in 5% of pregnancies. When the placenta was examined, 50% of the time they found bacteria associated with gum disease.

"What about the link between inflammation in the mouth and the whole body?"

This is the second part of the disease process. The body is naturally responding to the presence of bacteria. There are a few things that might happen.

At one end of the spectrum, the inflammation that is occurring in the mouth is limited and local. The overall constitution of the patient, their genetics, and their nutritional state are all favorable to resist the impact of the bacteria. Their body doesn't have other factors that would promote an exaggerated response. Their immune system mounts an appropriate response, and the bacteria might be held in check. Or they develop a localized problem that might involve slow bone deterioration over time.

"What about the other end of the spectrum?"

What we are recognizing is that many patients with periodontal disease will have an exaggerated response to the presence of bacterial plaque on their teeth. Here we will see that the presence of inflammation in the mouth will promote and exaggerate inflammation in the body and vice versa.

"What are the implications of this?"

An abundance of evidence shows correlations with chronic periodontal disease and many other health problems that are associated with inflammation.

Diseases such as heart disease, cancer of the colon, pancreas, and prostate have all been shown to have common links with periodontal disease. Diabetes and obesity, stroke, lung disease, kidney disease, the autoimmune diseases, and adverse outcomes of pregnancy have also been documented to have connections.

"What is causing the inflammation in the body?"

We are recognizing that there are common elements that promote systemic inflammation. Some people are predisposed because of genetics. We can't change our genes, though we can make choices in our lifestyle that influence how our genes are expressed.

As a result of the accumulation of toxins from outside sources—from eating foods that stress our bodies such as gluten, or from poor digestion—our bodies' metabolic pathways get bogged down. Our livers can become congested with a backlog of stuff it can't handle. We end up with an accumulation of waste products clogging the flow of lymph fluids from our tissues. Our immune systems react to all of this by trying to break it down to eliminate it. Because it is ongoing and the source doesn't get corrected, our immune systems get all fired up and are reacting non-stop.

When inflammation is occurring like this in our gum tissues, it ultimately causes breakdown of the tissues. Well, the same thing happens in other parts of our bodies as well. When the inflammation occurs within our joints, we experience arthritis. If in our blood vessels or heart valves, we experience cardiovascular disease.

"You had mentioned oxidative stress and free radicals?"

Our bodies need oxygen; however, it needs to be in balance. Too much of a concentration of oxygen can cause instability of important chemical compounds in the body. Much like what happens in a fire. Without oxygen, wood can't burn ... if you want it to burn faster you blow air or oxygen on it. If there is too much, a fire can rage out of control. This is what occurs with an excess of free radicals in the body; they act as a fire accelerant.

The unstable compounds caused by too much oxygen are called free radicals. They cause problems because of the chain reactions they cause, known as oxidative stress, which damages cell proteins, membranes, and genes, and contributes to systemic inflammation.

"How does chronic inflammation contribute to a disease like cancer?"

In a normal healthy condition, cells maintain a sense of their identity and relationship to their neighbors. They are in harmony with their environment outside of the cell. When the tissues surrounding the cells are in a state of chronic inflammation, there are numerous changes occurring that result in a change in the cell's perception. As described by cell biologist Bruce Lipton, a cell's perception is determined by the signals it gets from its environment and how it behaves in response to them.

Chronic inflammation changes the environment that our cells live in. As a result, the cells of the body can behave differently. Inflammation may lead to changes in the chemical environment both in the environment of cells as well as within them. This can lead to changes in the genes within the cells and lead to uncontrolled growth of the cells thus leading to tumors. Cells have lost their sense of belonging to the whole.

"So how does periodontal disease fit into this, and what can I do if I am concerned about the health of my gums?"

We know that proper treatment of the infection and inflammation of the gums will help to reduce inflammation within the body and improve one's general health.

For example, there are certain blood tests that a physician might use to detect signs of inflammation. A common test is called C reactive protein, or CRP. Studies have been done that show that thorough treatment of periodontal disease will lower levels of CRP and other blood indicators of inflammation in the body.

In a study published in the *New England Journal of Medicine* in 2007, it was found that thorough treatment of periodontitis resulted in improved blood flow in the brachial artery, a major artery that supplies blood to the lungs.

"Tells us about how periodontal disease is treated?"

There are various factors for us to consider. Good oral hygiene is essential, though other measures need to be taken to control and arrest gum disease.

Perhaps the most important of these is eliminating the bacteria that have been triggering the disease. This is done by a process of deep cleaning known as scaling and root planing that reduces the concentration of bacteria accumulated on the teeth and removes contaminants from the surfaces of the roots that have been deposited there by the bacteria. Often the biofilm that is created by the bacteria tends to return. In such cases, we will have the patient use a custom-fitted tray over their teeth with a peroxide gel that breaks down the stickiness of the plaque and keeps the film from reforming.

In advanced cases where the bacteria are embedded in the tissues, low doses of an antibiotic, doxycycline are used. Basically, it helps by inhibiting an enzyme that is created by the bacteria to help them invade the gum tissue.

The second is increasing the resistance of the individual patient to the disease. Here we look at lifestyle habits such as smoking and the patient's diet. We would also evaluate the patient for signs and symptoms of systemic inflammation, as well as acupuncture energy patterns that reflect toxicity and inflammation in the body.

There are general recommendations we will make for nutritional supplementation, as well as more specific recommendations based on the overall health of the patient. Often the patient will be referred to a nutritionist for assistance in determining their optimal diet.

"Tell us about some of the general nutritional guidelines?"

To start with, we would encourage the patient to shift their diet to a more plant-based, whole food diet. Meats should be eaten in moderation at best and should always be organic. One of the early pioneers in modern dentistry was Dr. Weston Price. He showed that people living in various parts of the world maintained good dental health with almost no tooth decay and gum disease when they ate a diet of whole foods that originated in their local environment. Whole foods being those foods usually found around the outer walls of most supermarkets where they sell produce, meats, fish, and dairy. (Actually, most dairy being pasteurized or heated to high temperatures would not be considered a whole food.)

It is important to be sure that most of what we eat be fruit or vegetables, to help maintain a healthy balance of our pH necessary to ensure proper mineral balance in the body.

"Why is that important?"

Researchers such as Harold Hawkins, DDS, and Melvin Page, DDS, found that to maintain bone health we need to maintain a ratio of calcium to phosphorous that is 10 to 4. If our diet is low in calcium or high in phosphorous, this balance can be thrown off and make us more susceptible to gum disease and tooth decay. Too much protein as well as carbonated beverages can lead to an excess of phosphorous and a relative deficiency of calcium. Leafy green vegetables are a good source of calcium. That's where cows get theirs.

"What are some of the specifics in nutrition and periodontal disease?"

It is essential to have adequate levels of vitamins.

First, if an individual has less than optimal nutritional intake of a nutrient like vitamin C, the gums will be less resistant to the invasive tendencies of the bacteria present. Vitamin C or ascorbic acid is used by the body in the synthesis of collagen—the major structural building block of the body's tissues. Historically, severe cases of vitamin C deficiency were seen in British sailors suffering from scurvy. Eventually, a cure was found by having them eat limes, which we now know are rich in vitamin C.

While many would benefit from more, as little as 500mg of vitamin C was shown to improve the health of the gums in a study at NYU's College of Dentistry.

Vitamin D has been found to have anti-inflammatory effects and may reduce susceptibility to gum disease. A study by Boston University evaluated the association between vitamin D status and gingivitis. They found that people with higher blood levels of vitamin D were less likely to experience bleeding gums.

"You spoke of oxidative stress and inflammation. What nutrients will help combat these in the battle against periodontal disease?"

A study published in the March 2009 issue of the *Journal of Periodontology* reveals that an antioxidant in green tea called catechin appears to reduce inflammation associated with periodontal disease. Antioxidants can reduce inflammation in the body, adding to growing evidence regarding the benefits of drinking green tea, especially in weight loss and control, heart health, and cancer prevention.

Curcumin, the active ingredient found in Turmeric, is known to exhibit many anti-inflammatory and health-promoting effects. In studies with rats, curcumin produced a significant reduction on the inflammatory infiltrate, and it increased collagen content and fibroblastic cell numbers. Curcumin potently inhibits innate immune responses associated with periodontal disease, suggesting a therapeutic potential in this chronic inflammatory condition.

There is some evidence linking gum disease to lower levels of coenzyme Q10, an antioxidant made naturally in the body, found widely in foods, and available in supplement form. Some researchers say that coenzyme Q10 is needed to properly repair gum tissue. A study by Osaka University in Japan found improvement in infection and inflammation after three weeks of using a topical coenzyme Q10 toothpaste.

Tea tree oil has proven antibiotic properties. A topically applied tea tree oil gel was evaluated in a double-blind placebo-controlled study involving 49 people with severe chronic gingivitis. They were told to brush twice a day and were assessed after four and eight weeks. The group that brushed with tea tree oil had a significant reduction in the degree of gingivitis and bleeding.

Conclusions

- Common dental disease such as tooth decay have plagued mankind for countless generations. It is clear from the evidence presented that these conditions are not merely conditions affecting the teeth but are intimately tied to our systemic health.

- Dental caries is primarily a condition associated with malnutrition and its effects on the biochemical integrity of the body. Diets that are grain based and include refined sugars support the growth of tooth decay promoting bacteria Strep Mutans in addition to shifting the biochemistry of the mouth to one that promotes tooth decay.

- Research into the relationships between periodontal disease and systemic illness is yielding a massive amount of information that provides a deeper understanding of the nature of disease in general, as well as the associations between systemic and oral health.

- Changes in the biological terrain of the body as a result of chronic malnutrition and toxicity promote inflammation and encourage changes in the biome of the body. This favors the degenerative process that occurs both with gum disease and associated degenerative diseases.

CHAPTER V
Our Physical Body and the Mouth

If the hip bone is connected to the knee bone, and the knee bone is connected to the ankle bone, what are the teeth and jaws connected to? Our whole body! That's right, our whole body.

It is time for "out of the box" thinking.

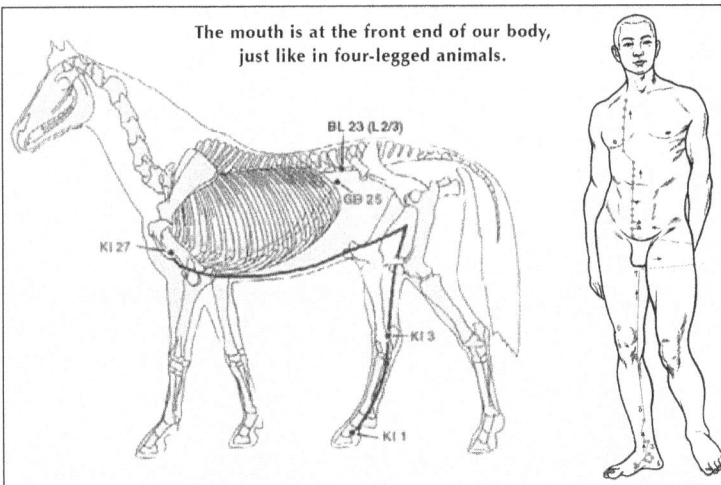

Figure 7: The meridians of man are similar to the other animals.

The bite (occlusion) of our teeth plays an integral role in the maintenance of the coordination and integration of function throughout our whole body. Having straight teeth that fit together properly promotes health and longevity. If this is not immediately evident to the reader, it is my intention to make it more so as you continue to read.

Many are affected by the influences of what dentists call malocclusion, or a bad bite. These influences may be subtle or more profound. Often, they are life changing and may be the cause, or a major contributing cause, of a diversity of symptoms. When problems are evident, the patient may be diagnosed as suffering from a temporomandibular disorder, also known as TMD or more commonly as "TMJ."

TMJ is often called "The Great Imposter" because the symptoms associated with it can be wide ranging, complicated, and difficult to relate to one another. Often, patients will have seen many doctors each treating the symptoms, but none recognizing the cause.

Common symptoms of TMJ may include headache, facial pain, and/ or neck pain, as well as any of the following:

- tension headaches
- migraines and other vascular headaches
- grinding or clenching of the teeth
- ear pain, otalgia
- ear ringing
- sinus pain or pressure
- ear stuffiness or pressure
- distorted hearing
- eye pain
- pain behind the eye, retro-orbital pain
- eye sensitivity
- back pain
- tender jaw muscles
- muscle tightness
- MPD or Myofascial Pain and Dysfunction
- fibromyalgia
- sleep disorders
- morning headaches
- muscle pain
- pain when biting, chewing, or yawning
- difficulties closing and opening the mouth
- popping or clicking sounds when opening the mouth
- sensitive teeth
- excessive tooth wear
- numbness in the fingers, hands, and arms
- and others

Fonder's Research on the Stress Caused by Bite Problems

In 1977, Aelred Fonder, DDS, published his book *The Dental Physician*. He described his clinical observations and research into the stress that is caused within the body as a result of malocclusion. Both he and a group of colleagues had spent years researching and documenting these effects.

He showed how the body would reflect many physical changes due to the stress of an imbalanced bite. Some physical changes were documented in three cases he treated that we share here, showing the posture and alignment of the body before and after his treatment. All three cases were treated by providing more balanced support for the bite by building up the patient's molar teeth with fillings.

A bite imbalance can often cause complex patterns of descending influences affecting body alignment and posture as seen in these three cases of spontaneous correction of scoliosis.

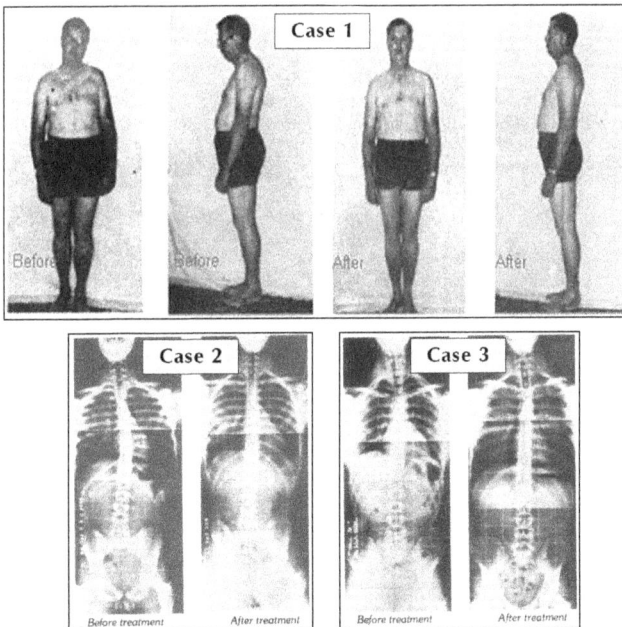

Figure 8: The alignment of the bite affects the alignment of the body

How is it that so many problems can be caused by a problem with my bite? To answer that, we need to understand more about the connections between the mouth and the body. First, a little bit about how our bite works.

How Do Teeth Work?

Each tooth is suspended in its socket by a pressure-sensing ligament that provides feedback to the central nervous system (CNS) and jaw muscles to regulate the forces and function of chewing and swallowing. Each tooth is designed for a different function and to bear a load in a different manner.

Our back teeth, the premolars and molars, are designed to support our jaw structure and associated muscles. They are designed with hills and valleys (cusps and fossa), designed to fit into one another so that the tops of hills on the upper teeth hit at the bottom of valleys on the lower teeth and vice versa. This allows the pressures of our bite to be transmitted directly along the roots of these teeth in a manner that promotes proper movement of the bones of our skull.

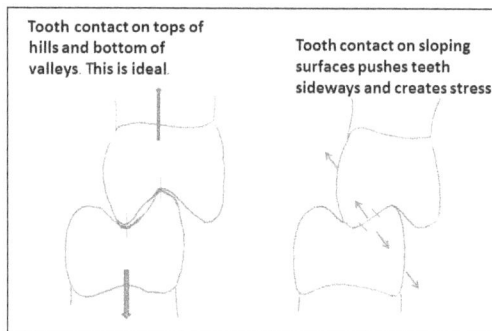

Figure 9: Author's depiction of bite forces acting on teeth after Dawson

The front teeth are designed to act like scissors to bite through and cut our food. They are designed so that the front edge of the lower incisor will slide across the contoured surface on the inner side of the upper incisors when we bite into our food. Much like the blades of a scissor, therefore the name <u>incisor</u>.

The teeth at the front corners known as <u>canines</u> (eye teeth) are designed to guide our jaws as we chew. This occurs in a very specific way that is profoundly related to maintaining the integrated function of the body from head to toe. When we chew, we open our mouth and can shift right or left to crush food between the back teeth. The canine teeth should be the first to contact causing our jaw to be guided back to center, the back teeth not actually meeting until the jaw is completely closed. Dentists call this "canine guidance."

Good "canine guidance" is important to the healthy function of the jaw, and it protects the other teeth from excessive wear. Nature's design is to limit the friction applied to our teeth when we chew. This will limit the wear on our teeth as well as promote the healthy function of our jaw. Unfortunately, varied events can interfere with the expression of nature's design and problems with the bite develop.

This function of the canine teeth in providing guidance is related to the muscles that open and move the jaw sideways. These are called the **Lateral Pterygoid** (pronounced ter-goid) muscles. It is common to see problems in the function of these muscles as a consequence of the canine teeth not being in the correct position. This results in problems of coordination of the muscle, as well as increased tension in the muscle. The consequences can be profound as the effects ripple through the body.

These muscles originated on the side of wings of a bone that extends down from the base of the skull behind our eyes. This is called the sphenoid bone. The muscle then extends back-

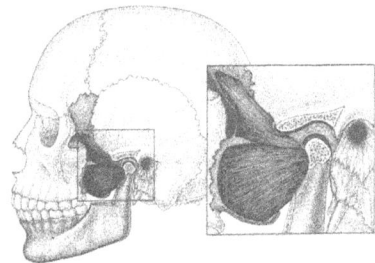

Figure 10: Illustration of Lateral Pterygoid muscle
From Travell & Simons' *Myofascial Pain & Dysfunction: The Trigger Point Manual*
With permission from the publisher

ward and to the side to attach to the jawbone at the jaw joint.

When the Lateral Pterygoid muscle is in chronic tension because of poor position or form of the canine (eye) tooth, it will pull on the base of the skull. The bone it pulls on is the sphenoid bone. It interferes with its movement and often affects its position. The sphenoid bone is like a keystone in the architecture of the skull. If it doesn't function correctly, all is affected.

It is known in chiropractic and osteopathy that the movements of the sphenoid are mirrored by the movements of the sacrum (the bone that sits in the middle of our pelvis). Distortions of the sphenoid position or movement are reflected in the sacrum and pelvis.

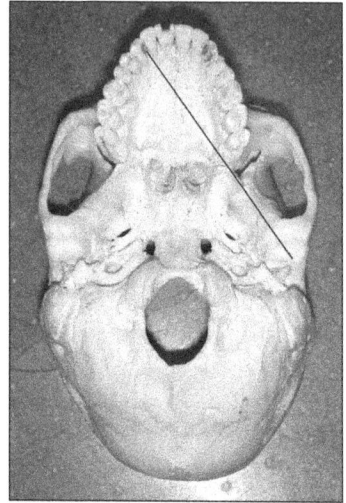

Figure 11: The Lateral Pterygoid muscle, as well as other jaw muscles, can develop tension when they are overworked and not allowed to come to rest. This happens when the bite is poorly developed and doesn't guide the jaw to a relationship that supports the muscles at their proper length. More on this to be discussed below.

Along with these imbalances in the bones, there are concurrent influences through the musculoskeletal chains of the meridians so that disruptions in the jaw muscles are reflected along the kinetic pathways of the meridians in other parts of the body.

Improper canine guidance is responsible for different effects within the body. Frequently lack of canine guidance will be responsible for the instability of muscles in the low back and waist, resulting in pelvic torsions that result in one leg appearing shorter than the other and leading to low back pain. There is a specific muscle, the psoas, which is directly influenced by poor function of the lateral pterygoid muscle. This can be demonstrated using the methods of Applied Kinesiology, which is described below and in more depth in Chapter VI, "How We Know What Is Going On."

More on How the Bite Can Affect the Rest of the Body: The Physical Connections of the Mouth

My introduction to a holistic understanding of the mouth (stomatognathic system) began in 1980 with an eighteen-month association working in the office of Dr. Harold Gelb. He stimulated my interest in looking at the interrelationships between the mouth (stomatognathic system) and the body as a whole. I began to learn about the **potential for stress being created in the body when there was a misalignment of the jaw and/or bite (occlusal) disharmony.**

Dr. Gelb also introduced me to the work of Dr. George Goodheart, who was the father of the clinical science of **Applied Kinesiology**. Kinesiology is the study of the body's movement and the mechanisms by which it occurs. Applied Kinesiology is essentially the practice of applying this knowledge to optimize body function.

Applied Kinesiology can teach us much about the relationships that exist between the mouth (stomatognathic system) and the rest of the body. When we dissect the muscles of the body, they appear separate. In fact, they exist as integral components of our neuromuscular system. They never function without the influence of other muscles (agonists and antagonists). The whole of our body's nervous and muscular system is in constant interplay. As a consequence, dysfunction of a jaw (masticatory) muscle has the potential to disrupt the function of muscles quite removed anatomically.

This has been nicely demonstrated by studies that have shown increased tension within lower back muscles when a bite interference is introduced to the molars. It is also borne out by a study of acupuncture energetics from a neuromuscular point of view. Further evidence is seen daily by me and fellow practitioners who are prepared by training and experience.

The alignment of the jaw structures at rest and the contacts of teeth during chewing and swallowing have a profound impact on the functioning of the body as a whole. The use of Applied Kinesiology permits us to disclose when a disruptive influence is present within the stomatognathic (mouth-chewing) system. In association with other diagnostic tools, Applied Kinesiology can be used to localize the problem and define it. It can also be used in combination with our other clinical skills to correct the source of dysfunction. More about Applied Kinesiology will be explored in Chapter VI.

During that period in the early eighties, I had the opportunity to study with Mariano Rocabado, RPT, a physical therapist from Chile. He had just begun to teach other physical therapists and dentists about the **orthopedic and neuromuscular relationships of the head and neck**.

He discussed how improper posture of the head and neck could come about as a result of mouth breathing and nasal obstruction associated with allergies in kids. This would lead to mouth breathing and poor muscle function of the tongue during swallowing. He also spoke about the **need to correct the patient's posture in the process of determining the correct relationship between the lower jaw (mandible) and its craniofacial articulations.**

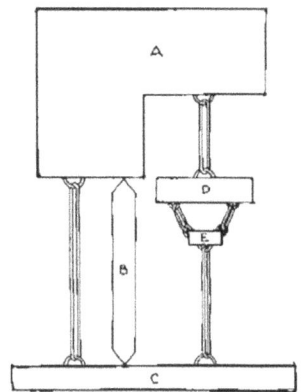

Figure 12: This diagram represents the muscle support of the head and neck.

The head (A) is balanced on the vertebral column (B), and shoulder girdle (C), with the lower jaw (D) and hyoid bone(E) connected by muscles depicted by elastics on the front and back of the neck.
From Current Advances in Dentistry, Telephone Extension Program, University of Illinois College of Dentistry 1949

Postural Balance of the Head and Neck Is Profoundly Affected by Complex Interactions with Jaw Alignment and the Bite of the Teeth

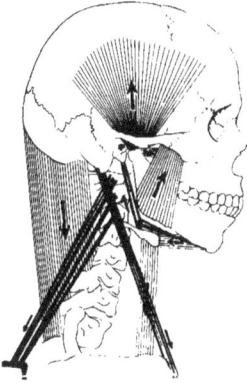

Figure 13: In this diagram, we can see that the lower jaw is suspended from the head and is a link in the chain of muscles at the back, sides, and front of the head and neck.

Misalignment of the teeth results in misalignment of the jaws, resulting in alteration to the posture of the head and neck.

This lady is missing an upper and lower incisor resulting in her other teeth being in an improper position that affects the function of her jaw and neck muscles when she chews.

As she moves her mouth to chew, we can see tension develop in the muscles of her neck. This is not normal.

While attending Rocabado's lecture, I was sitting next to another physical therapist named John Barnes, RPT. We became friends. John was engaged in the development and teaching of a therapy he called Myofascial Release. This innovative therapy dealt with restrictions that occurred in the soft tissues of the body due to poor habits, chronic tension, stress, and injury.

I attended a number of workshops that John offered which would help me understand and develop some skill in his approach. John had recognized that many people develop chronic tension in their muscles and, in turn, the connective tissues that give our body form and hold

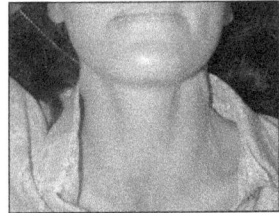

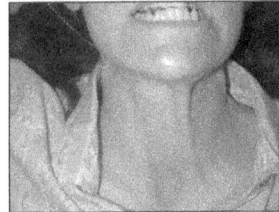

us together. Over time, this tension would cause changes that would restrict the body's flexibility and free movement, and result in chronic pain. John evolved unique techniques using manual therapy and gentle stretching to counter the tension in the tissues that would restore their flexibility.

Around the same time, I had the good fortune to be introduced to the concepts of osteopathic medicine. Initially, I studied the work of Dr. John E. Upledger, an osteopathic physician. He practiced in a specialized field of osteopathic manual medicine and developed his own unique approach he called CranioSacral Therapy. The Upledger Institute offers training that is unparalleled in the hands-on diagnosis and treatment of the connective tissue system of the body. I subsequently have received training from other osteopathic physicians to further develop my palpatory and manual skills in cranial osteopathy.

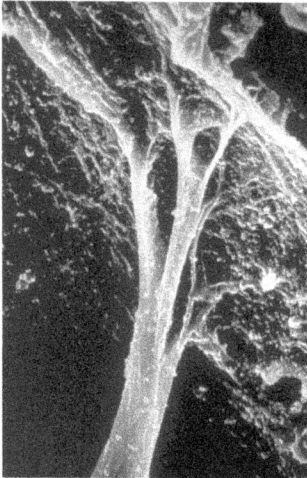

Figure 14: Connective tissue within the sutures of the skull
Copyright Image courtesy of Upledger Institute International /John E. Upledger's Cranial and Intracranial Membrane Image and Series

When the body is viewed from a physical perspective, we see that all of the body's organs and tissues are supported and held together by the connective tissue system.

These tissues are continuous from head to toe, from the skin to the core of our nervous system, from the most macroscopic perspective to the most microscopic.

The tissues that compose these pathways include all of the body's tissues and fluids.

These structures form chains of muscles, fascia, skeletal components, and organs creating the body's structural-kinetic pathways.

The image above is of connective tissue within the suture of a human skull. This connective tissue is continuous with all of the body tissue.

Cranial Osteopathy and Dentistry

As a student at Temple University School of Dentistry, I was taught that the function of the sutures in the skull was to permit growth and expansion of the cranial vault, and at some point, after growth and development had been completed, the sutures would fuse together.

What I didn't know at the time was that these conclusions about the purpose of cranial sutures were based on the study of cadaver (dead bodies) material and had little basis in fact. It comes as a surprise to many dentists to find out that what we were taught in dental school about the "ossification" of cranial sutures isn't really so.

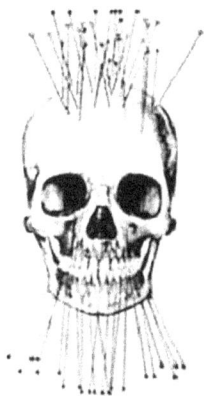

Figure 15: Depiction of the force vectors generated by the bite being absorbed in the skull; from Dempsey circa 1941

Though our skull may seem rigid, it is pliable and made of 22 bones that move in relation to one another. In a state of health, cranial sutures are lined with elastic connective tissues that permit subtle, yet definite movements to occur. The bones of the skull are designed to fit in an ingenious way to permit expansion and contraction. This has been known for many years within the chiropractic and osteopathic professions and was initially brought to light by the work of Sutherland in the early 1900s.

As we bite, the forces generated are transmitted along the roots of the teeth and pass into the bones of the skull. When the jaw is aligned and the bite balanced, the forces directed into the skull are dissipated in a manner that supports healthy function of the cranial mechanism. Problems with the bite will cause distortion in the shape and movement of these bones.

This affects what is known as the craniosacral system, an essential part of body function, which involves the meningeal (dural) membranes as a functional link between the physiologic micro-motion of the bones of the cranium and pelvis.

The dural membranes lining the skull contain a semi-closed hydraulic system designed to facilitate the flow of cerebrospinal fluid. As such, the craniosacral system is a physiological system. These dural membranes are attached to the inside (internal periosteum) of the cranial bones and to the second and third vertebrae but are unattached as they pass through the spinal column—until the tailbone (sacrum) is reached. Once again, there is a firm attachment.

This photo shows the dural membranes that line the skull dividing the space, providing support to the brain, and providing connections via the dural tube of the spinal cord to the sacrum and pelvis. Movements of bones within the skull are mirrored by movements within the tailbone (sacrum).

Figure 16: The membranes within the skull
Copyright Image courtesy of Upledger Institute International /John E. Upledger's Cranial and Intracranial Membrane Image and Series

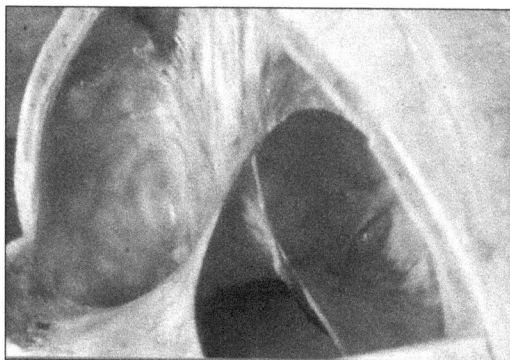

The Meningeal Membranes:

The meningeal dural tube is viewed as the "core link" connecting the occiput and the sacrum.

With balance, the occiput and sacrum move normally.

A balanced bite of the teeth is essential to support balance within the cranial-sacral system

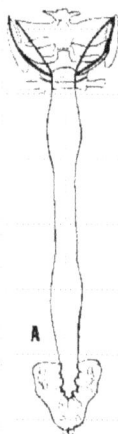

Figure 17: This picture illustrates the skull at the top and the sacrum at the bottom, connected by the dural tube.

A strain in the skull caused by a dental bite problem will affect the dural tube and balance of the sacrum.

from *Craniopathy and Dentistry* by David G Denton, DC self published 1979

64

Understanding the craniosacral system is important when it comes to understanding and treating many cases with temporomandibular dysfunction (TMD). For example, when there is a strain within the pelvis, there will be a corresponding strain within the cranial system that can contribute to TMJ symptoms. Which came first the chicken or the egg? As Dr. Upledger used to say, it is important to take a whole body approach in diagnosis and treatment of TMJ problems.

The Myofascial Meridian Pathways

During the period 1995-1996, I enrolled in the Physician/Dentist Acupuncture certification program at Tri-State Institute in New York City. The founder of the school, Mark Seem, Ph.D., developed what he calls a system of "American acupuncture." In this approach to acupuncture, recognition is given to the fact that when acupuncture needles are being placed, they are inserted into these myofascial connective tissues.

In the meridian approach to acupuncture treatment taught at Tri-State Institute, the patient's complaints are used as a guide in the palpatory examination of the patient's myofascial connective tissues. The clinician seeks to locate areas of tightness and tension that are signs of restricted energy flow. These areas may be experienced as tender or painful by the patient. In the Japanese style of acupuncture, these points are called ashi or kori. When painful, they are described as trigger points in Western terminology.

In the meridian approach, these areas of energy blockage manifesting as tight and tender points are sites at which treatment is applied, usually with needles. In conjunction with this local treatment to the areas that are painful, treatment is applied to distal points in the hands and feet to facilitate the relaxation of the zone being treated.

Eliminating tight tender areas restores normal physiology and flow of energy to the affected myofascial tissues, thus eliminating pain and promoting balance of the body. This is particularly critical in under-standing the whole body influence of malocclusion.

As we examine the pathways of energy movement in the body, we see these pathways flow down (Yang) from the jaws and the head, down the neck and shoulders and the back of the hands and arms, along the back, side and front of the body as they pass through the legs and ankles to the toes where they turn around and run their course from the ground up (Yin) through the inner parts of the legs, and up through the torso.

As the meridians pass through the head, coursing through the brain, the fascia, the cranial bones, the muscles, the jaws, and the teeth, they are subject to the effect of distortions within the cranial mechanism (the bones of the skull and the connective tissues attached to them that facil-itate their inherent motion).

A misalignment of the bite will produce changes structurally, functionally, and energetically through the muscles, the cranial-sacral sytem, and the meridians; all is one.

Axis of Gravity

Distorted Plane
of Occlusion

Scoliosis of
the Spine

Unstable
Pelvis

Collapse of the
joints of the
Feet & Ankles

Figure 18: *From Physiologic Occlusion* by James Carlson, DDS
with permission from the author

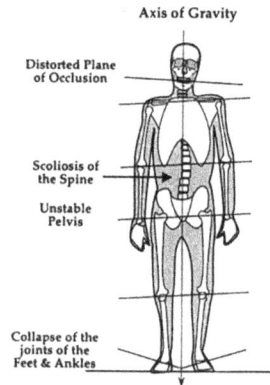

Distortion and strain within the cranial mechanism are often caused by misalignment of the jaws and imbalance in the distribution of biting forces acting on the teeth.

The maldistribution of forces of the bite due to missing teeth, improper replacement of teeth, or malocclusion will impact on the bio-mechanics of the skull and be reflected throughout the myofascial and musculotendinous meridian systems.

An example of this was seen in a patient of mine, Lynne G.

CASE REPORT: Lynne G. presented for dental treatment, requiring a crown to be placed on her upper right molar to restore it. The tooth had previously been treated with root canal therapy, at which time it had been shortened to take biting pressure off it. About a month after we had placed a provisional acrylic crown, Lynne called me to report that she had an amazing experience. The heel of her right foot had been giving her a burning intermittent pain for two years. As soon as we placed this temporary crown on this tooth, the pain disappeared. In fact, it stayed away for four weeks only to return that morning after the temporary crown came loose from her tooth.

Using Applied Kinesiology, I evaluated the causal chain between her foot pain and her tooth. It seems that the absence of support for the bite on this tooth was permitting a slight torquing of the mandible when she closed her mouth. This in turn was interfering with the micro-motion of the bilateral maxillary bones and at the same time inducing a torsion of the sphenobasilar junction. It was fascinating to see the meridian energetic influences generated by this dental cranial stress. Both the Bladder meridian and Triple Warmer reacted kinesiologically throughout their entire course, as if the energy transmitted along them was blocked.

As soon as I replaced the temporary crown and re- evaluated the cranial and meridian indicators they were completely non- reactive. The pain she had suffered was completely dissipated.

Continuing my education, I studied with Dr. Phillipe Druelle, an osteopath from Canada. He taught about the fascial relationships between the organs and the rest of the body. He trained us to palpate the organs and their inherent motion, to distinguish between normal and constrained movement. He taught us how to treat what was abnormal, supporting the body in healing itself.

Subsequently, I observed that this constraint in the movement of organs would be reflected through the associated acupuncture meridian with signs of tension and constraint of energy. This can readily be mapped out in the body by the use of Applied Kinesiology testing. I developed a method of mapping out the stress vectors along the myofascial meridians some time later.

CASE REPORT: A Dental Connection to a Sleep Disturbance

This is illustrated by a case involving a patient named Nadine. She was having trouble sleeping. She was awakening every night about 3 o'clock a.m. In Chinese medicine, it is understood that our organ systems are dominant at different times of the 24-hour daily cycle. When we sleep, our liver has time to catch up with the myriad of tasks it has to complete. The Liver/ Gall Bladder meridian is dominant at 3:00 a.m.

Nadine's chiropractor was expert in providing her with nutritional guidance. Despite all efforts to support the liver, Nadine's sleep disturbance continued. She came to see me for a consultation. What I found was there were imperfections with her bite that were causing certain teeth to hit on inclined planes instead of tops of hills and bottoms of valleys. Remember we discussed this before. It is a source of stress.

The result was a strain within the myofascial meridians connecting her upper jaw in the area of these teeth to the Liver/ Gall Bladder meridians.

Correcting the problem with her bite by doing fine adjustments to the shape of the affected teeth and relieving the excessive noxious pressure led to resolution of the tension within the meridian and a normalization of the energy flow. Her sleep problem resolved.

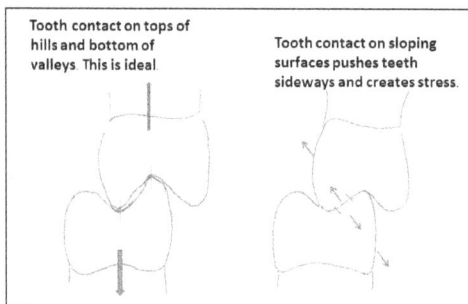

Tooth contact on tops of hills and bottom of valleys. This is ideal.

Tooth contact on sloping surfaces pushes teeth sideways and creates stress.

Figure 19: Author's depiction of bite forces acting on teeth after Dawson

Bite Problems Can Affect the Rhythm of Your Heart

A disturbance of the muscles of the neck, shoulder, and chest is often associated with poor occlusion (bite). This results in the development of some tension and soreness in a major chest muscle called the pectoralis major. There is a specific area in this muscle along the lower border of the chest bone where a trigger point can develop. This has been associated by Janet Travel, M.D. and other researchers with cardiac arrhythmia. Pain from this trigger point will often be mistaken for heart pain. Many of the patients we see with this problem complain of feeling anxious.[19]

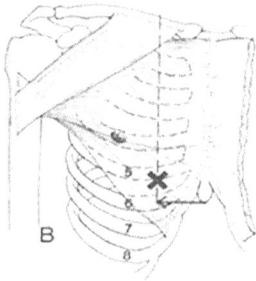

Figure 20: From Travell & Simons'
Myofascial Pain & Dysfunction:
The Trigger Point Manual
With permission from the publisher

In the diagram above, the **X** marks the trigger point that Dr. Janet Travel, MD described as the "cardiac arrhythmia" trigger point. She described it as being on the lower border of the fifth rib in the vertical line that lies midway between the sternal margin and the nipple line.

This point **X** corresponds to the acupuncture point Kidney 22.

Evaluation of the energy flow in the meridians will reveal an excess of energy (over stimulation) in the heart channel and a deficiency (weakness) in the kidney channel. If using Applied Kinesiology to test the strength of the pectoralis major, it will be weak.

Therapy localization (testing a strong muscle while bringing attention to an area of suspected stress) to the trigger points described above

---

19. *The Dental Connection in Cardiac Pain and Arrhythmia*, by David Lerner, DDS poster presentation at the Annual Scientific meeting of the American Academy of Cranio-facial Pain.

will cause a strong muscle to weaken. Therapy localization to a point on the kidney channel (K3) on the opposite foot will also cause a strong muscle to weaken. However, contacting this kidney point (K3) on the opposite foot (or placing an acupuncture needle) will cause the weak pectoralis major to strengthen. Until the patient bites down and moves the jaw side to side, then all will be undone again. Providing proper support and guidance to the bite will resolve this problem. It is important that, if deficient, the shape of the eyeteeth is corrected so that they are able to provide the dominant contact when the jaw shifts to the side during chewing. The entire syndrome will resolve and the chest tension will disappear, as will the anxiety. Case closed.

CASE REPORT: We treated a woman who had been suffering from a heart rhythm irregularity that could not be explained by the physicians she had consulted. She traveled the country searching for an answer until ending up in the office of an integrative physician in St. Louis that was familiar with our work. When he found she lived within an hour drive from our office, he suggested she see us for a dental evaluation.

Over the years, she had had a lot of dental work with crowns and bridges placed on many of her teeth. Her bite had progressively been thrown off balance resulting in the syndrome described above. We first treated her with a specific type of appliance to correct the alignment of her jaw and balance her bite. Her symptoms quickly resolved. Subsequently, we replaced her defective crowns and bridgework to provide a permanent result.

Bite Problems Will Affect the Lower Back

The bite is also a contributing factor in many cases with low back pain and short leg syndrome. This occurs as a result of the tension occurring in the lateral pterygoid muscle (the jaw opening muscle), which in turn pulls at the sphenoid bone (makes up the front part of the bottom of the

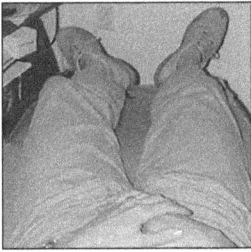

Figure 21: The patient's left leg is rotated outward due to weakness of the Psoas muscle resulting from poor function of the Lateral Pterygoid muscle of the jaw.

skull) upsetting the balance within the cranio-sacral mechanism.

A common observation in this scenario is that a major muscle of the low back, the psoas, becomes weak. As the psoas weakens, other muscles in the low back become tense in response and begin to pull up on the pelvic bone (ilium) on this side.

The net result is that the hip is pulled higher on the side where the leg appears to be shorter. This is called a functional short leg to distinguish from the more uncommon occurrence when there is an anatomical discrepancy in the length of leg bones (an anatomically short leg).

Another sign that the psoas is weakened is that when the patient is lying on their back, their leg will rotate out, causing their toes to point out instead of to the ceiling.

Problems originating elsewhere on the body impacting the cranio-sacral system can lead to symptoms of facial and jaw pain. In these cases, dental intervention may be contraindicated. A bite plate or occlusal adjustment may worsen the patient's condition if applied at the wrong time. Often, it is better if the patient is first treated to relieve myofascial tension that has accumulated and their system brought into a better state of relaxation.

Teeth and How They Keep Us from Falling Down

How do we stand up without falling down? As Buckminster Fuller described it, like all natural structures, our body may be described as a tensegrity system. In such a system, there is a balance of forces of tension and compression.

Think of a circus tent with the vertical poles supporting the weight of

the canvas, and ropes tied to stakes in the ground gen-
erating tension that balances the weight of the canvas
over the poles. In simple terms, we might say that
the weight of our body is resting on and supported
by our skeletal system, and our muscles, tendons,
and ligaments generate a tension that is equal on the
front, sides, and back of the body thus balancing us on our skeleton.

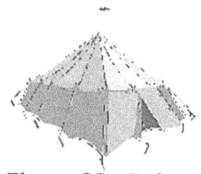

Figure 22: A circus tent is held up by tensegrity

If we were to consider this phenomenon of the tensegrity of the body
from the perspective of acupuncture energetics, we would see that this
concept can be described in terms of the Chinese medical concepts of Yin
and Yang. When the posture of the body is correct, there will be a relaxed
and balanced tension within our muscles and the horizontal planes of our
body will be parallel and at right angles to the long axis of the body. This
facilitates the maintenance of the structural and functional organization.
This state promotes health. Nature's forces are in a state of equilibrium
with the Yin and Yang forces acting on the body in equilibrium. Distortions
in the bite and plane of occlusion are reflected throughout the body.

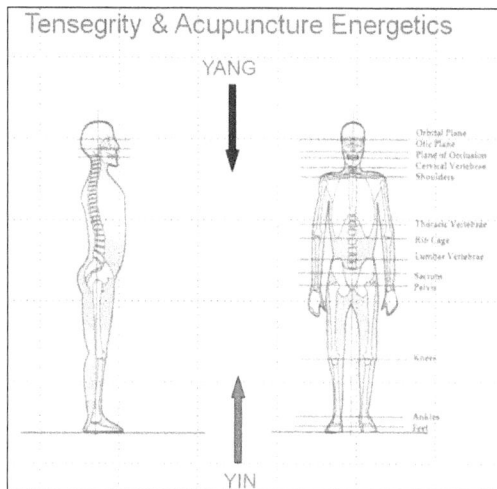

Figure 23: The body is supported by the balance of the forces of Yin and Yang
illustration adapted from *Physiologic Occlusion* by James Carlson DDS

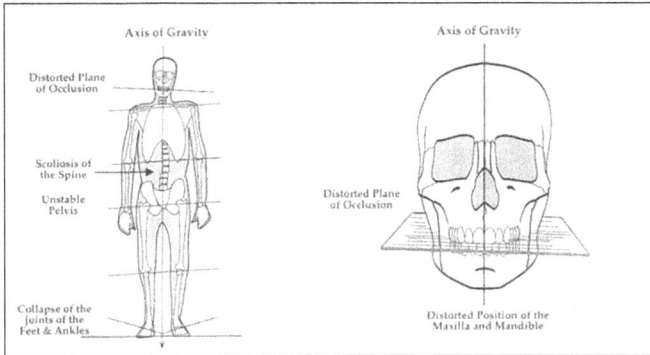

**Figure 24: Illustrations from *Physiologic Occlusion*,
by James E. Carlson, DDS**
used with permission from the author

Growth and development gone wrong develop common patterns of distortion. Let's look at a couple of common patterns of distortion: somato visceral causative chains.

A misalignment of the jaw to the side will produce changes structurally, functionally, and energetically through the muscles, the craniosacral mechanism, and the meridians. The body is one.

There will be a predominant influence on the descending channel of Gall Bladder and the ascending Liver channel. The skull will be constrained on the side that the mandible has deviated to as well as the Gall Bladder meridian. This predisposes the patient to torsion patterns of the craniosacral system and disequilibrium.

CASE REPORT: An example of what happens when the forces acting on the bite and cranial system are severely off balance is presented in the case of Carol. Carol suffered from chronic pain as well as difficulty walking which had arisen over time. Her sense of disequilibrium was so bad that Carol had to lean against a wall or some other stationary object as she walked.

When looking at her leg length when she was lying on her back, there was a significant discrepancy apparent in the length of her legs.

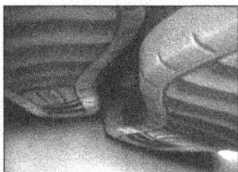

Carol's right leg appeared about an inch shorter than her left.

When looking at Carol's face from the front, the lack of symmetry is obvious.

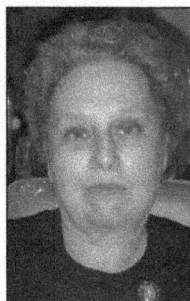

Her lower jaw shifted to the right and her bite over closed on this side, causing her face to be shorter on this side.

This resulted in a lack of muscular symmetry and balance throughout her body.

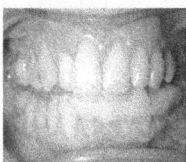

We initially treated Carol with a sectional bite support to allow the correct alignment of her jaw and other cranial bones.

As we fitted this sectional appliance to balance the forces within her skull, Carol's sense of disequilibrium improved.

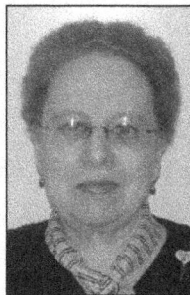

After a couple of months of chiropractic care and fine-tuning of the appliance, her face became symmetrical.

And her leg lengths became even.

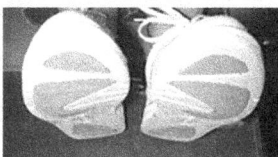

Another classical pattern of imbalance will be seen with a retruded jaw. In this pattern, there will also be changes structurally, functionally, and energetically throughout the muscles, the craniosacral mechanism, and the meridians.

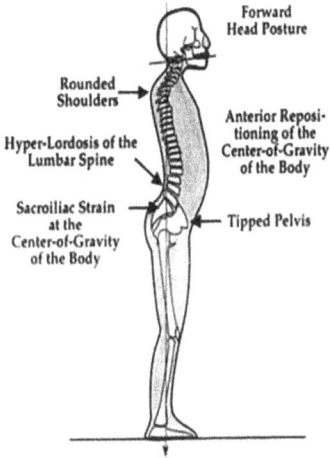

Forward
Head Posture

Rounded
Shoulders

Hyper-Lordosis of the
Lumbar Spine

Anterior Reposi-
tioning of the
Center-of-Gravity
of the Body

Sacroiliac Strain
at the
Center-of-Gravity
of the Body

Tipped Pelvis

Figure 25: There will be a predominant influence on the descending (*Yang*) Bladder meridian and the ascending (*Yin*) Kidney meridian.

The muscles along the Bladder channel in the back will tend to be more tense, resisting and/or reacting to the changes in the posture of the head on the neck.

Chronic stress reactions within the body resulting from unfavorable body mechanics will contribute to adrenal fatigue, manifesting as kidney deficiencies.

The influence observed follows a precept laid down thousands of years ago in *The Yellow Emperor's Classic of Internal Medicine*, "*as Yang tends to excess, Yin tends towards deficiency.*"

The structural imbalances often seen with malocclusion often result in strain and tension within the myofascial systems of the body in a manner that affects the balanced flow of energy. The patterns of stress within the body can be mapped out using Applied Kinesiology as described below.

Dental-Somatic Stress Vector Analysis

Over the years working with Applied Kinesiology and my understanding of the cranial sacral system and the acupuncture meridians, I developed a method of analysis of the strains and restrictions within the body that resulted from, or were associated with, malocclusion of the teeth. This is done by observing the posture of the patient, muscle palpation, and mostly by evaluating strain patterns within the myofascia that could be demonstrated by Applied Kinesiology.

The muscle testing response is observed as meridians are palpated and the skin connected to the underlying myofascia is challenged by light tensions applied with finger pressure. Lines with arrows are drawn to show direction of strain and x's are marked where there are areas of muscle tension as shown below.

CASE REPORT: The patient had prior orthodontic treatment with a lack of symmetry created in the arch form as seen in the photo of her upper teeth. She has a scoliosis with the left shoulder elevated and slightly rotated forward. Her left ear is more prominent than the right as the bones holding the ears are not in sync with one another. She had been suffering headaches and had a recent bout with Bell's palsy which had resolved.

Figure 26: A diagram showing the lines of stress through the patient's body. A Stress Vector Diagram

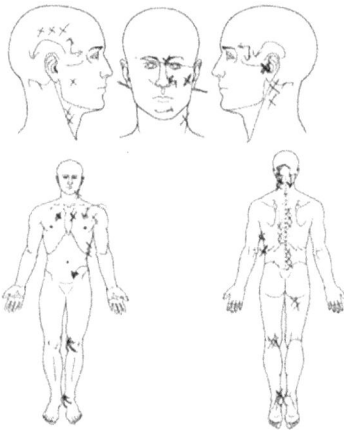

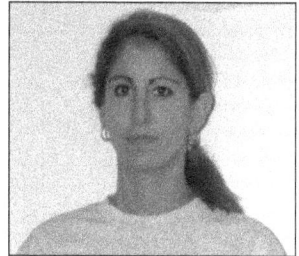

Figure 27 above and 28 below: Note the asymmetry in the patient's face and body.

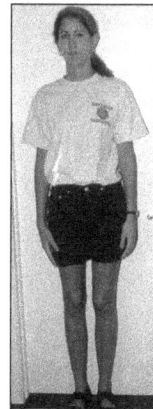

Figure 29: Note the asymmetry in the patient's upper jaw

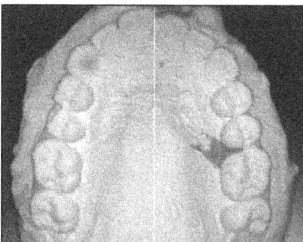

Figuring Things Out

It's important for a dentist to know what is correct for a given patient's bite. The teeth need to meet in such a way as to properly transfer the forces of biting and chewing so that the structures of the skull can function properly. The jaw muscles must be functioning in an environment that permits full relaxation when at rest to permit maintenance of proper muscle tone. This is essential for proper postural support of the head, neck, shoulder girdle, etc.

Ultimately, the proof is in the pudding, so to speak. Is the patient comfortable? However, because of the myriad of influences within the body, the patient often can't tell what is right, especially when they have not had the experience of "right" for an extended time. That's why dentists need a method to evaluate the patient's bite and determine if it is healthy or not.

There are schools of thought, as well as thoughtful dentists, evolving in the right direction. Mostly the methods treat the mouth as an independent system of the body, not appreciating or respecting the impact the treatments may have on the body as a whole. The predominant schools of thought are the concepts of Centric Relation and Neuromuscular Dentistry. I will discuss these and then share my philosophy and approach to treatment.

Centric Relation

First, let's discuss the philosophy of **Centric Relation**. This term describes a condition where the structures within the TM joint are in a normal relationship. In a sense, the TM joint itself is then used as a reference point from which the bite is figured out. This method may work well in the hands of a well-trained dentist, though not always as we shall see. One of the most well-known advocates of this method is the Dawson Academy, which promotes the life work of Dr. Peter Dawson.

Dr. Dawson who is in his mid-eighties as of this writing has been a thought leader that has promoted the need to be more aware of the relationship between the bite of the teeth and the jaw joint.

In my experience, I have had much success using what I have learned from the Dawson Academy. The principles taught are foundational to providing a high level of technical, functional, and aesthetic excellence in the restorative dentistry we provide to our patients. The methods taught are valuable for diagnosing what is wrong with a patient's bite and planning how to correct the problem. These principles have been very helpful in resolving chronic jaw clenching and tooth grinding in many of our patients.

The dentist must be trained to evaluate the joint relationship, and when a misalignment is observed, guide the jaw and joint relationship to a corrected alignment. This can be very subjective however, due to changes that can occur within the tissues of the joint in response to mechanical stresses, as well as, the dentist's understanding of what is normal joint physiology, and their skills in guiding the jaw to correct joint alignment.

I have treated many patients with these methods that have had relief from headaches and other complaints as well. A significant number of others have not. As advanced as these methods are, they are not complete. They do not measure or consider the role of the neuromuscular system and its relation to dental occlusion.

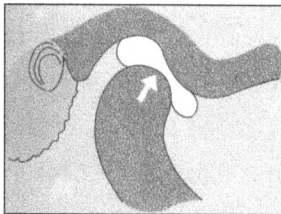

Figure 30: This drawing
shows the normal
relationship of structures
in the TM joint.

Below is a photo of a dissected normal joint:

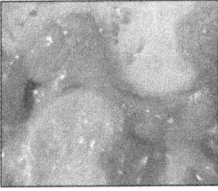

And a Cone Beam image of a normal joint:

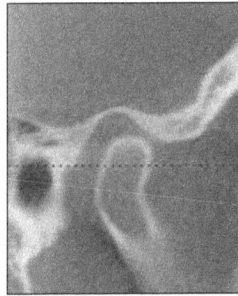

But what about when the joint looks like this:

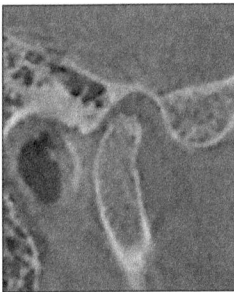

Jaw retruded

Or this:

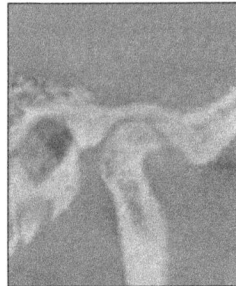

**Jaw retruded and over closed
vertically with reactive
overgrowth of condyle**

The methods of Centric Relation are focused on the jaw joint and do not measure or evaluate for neuromuscular dysfunction. Therefore, correction of associated neuromuscular problems is hit or miss. When the patient doesn't get better the doctor may conclude there is something "wrong" with the patient and not the treatment. There is a need for a more comprehensive physiologic approach that allows us to understand and correct the underlying imbalance of the neuromuscular function of our patients.

What about the Plasticity of Joint Anatomy and Condylar Remodeling?

It has also been shown that the structures of the TM joint will become deformed because of an inappropriate load being placed on it due to lack of support from the bite. This is seen in the image above to the right with reactive overgrowth of the condyle. The lack of proper support can be the result of an injury, poor childhood development, incorrect orthodontic treatment, the loss of teeth, or improper repair and replacement of teeth.

There are challenges presented when the structures in the joint are misplaced and may have degenerated, in such conditions how do we determine the "normal" relationship or Centric Relation? The answer lies in taking a broader perspective and evaluating the health and balance of the muscles involved in jaw posture and function.

NEUROMUSCULAR DENTISTRY: Using technology to assist in diagnosis and correction of the bite and re-establishment of neuromuscular harmony

Neuromuscular dentistry is an approach to diagnosis and correction of bite disorders that make use of computerized measurements of the function of the jaw and neck muscles as well as the movements of the jaw and TM joint.

This technology developed through the combined effort of a dentist, Dr. Bernard Jankelson, and an engineer, John Radke. Their approach was based on the belief that if they first relaxed the jaw muscles, it would be easier to find the correct position of the bite. They based their work on principles originally developed by Dr. Janet Travel, a pioneer in the treatment of chronic pain.

Their goal was to resolve the pain and tension in the muscles of the jaw by first relaxing the muscles using an electronic device called a TENS (trans-cutaneous electrical nerve stimulator). They developed instruments and methods that allow measurements to be made and recorded by a computer, providing insight into the muscular imbalances being caused by the bite. Then, using an appliance worn on the teeth to correct the form of the bite, the jaw would "reposition" to the most relaxed and comfortable position.

There are different components to the systems that have evolved that are now manufactured by two different companies, Myotronics (a company developed by Jankelson) and Bioresearch (a company developed by Radke).

The first of these is **EMG,** or electromyography, which has been widely used in physical medicine. This uses small pads applied to the skin over key jaw muscles connected to a computer by wires. The greater the tension that is present in the muscle, the higher the output of electrical impulses picked up by the computer will be. This gives much insight into the influence of the bite as a cause of muscular imbalance and pain.

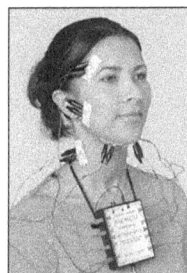

Figure 31: A patient set up for EMG measurement of the jaw muscles

EMG allows us to observe lack of symmetry and balance in the jaw muscles. Measurements are made of the muscles at rest and in function. When the bite is correct the muscles are able to relax, and when the patient lightly closes their teeth together in their bite, the muscles will stay relaxed. If the jaw has to shift for the teeth to fit, or if they don't fit properly, the muscles will develop tension.

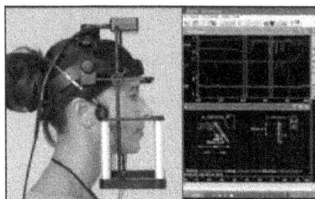

Figure 32: The Jaw Tracker used to measure movements of the jaw

The second key element is the **Jaw Tracker** which measures the movements of the jaw. One very important movement that is measured is how the jaw moves from a position where the muscles are relaxed to a position where all the teeth are biting together.

With a healthy bite and muscular relationship, a reference point on the front teeth will move a short distance of about 1.5-2mm on a straight lineup and slightly forward as the jaw closes from rest. When there is a neuromuscular imbalance created by the bite, the jaw will have to shift from its relaxed position, often moving backwards and to the side as the muscles contract unevenly to get the bite to fit together.

As the jaw shifts on closure as a result of an ill-fitting bite, the TM joint is affected. As the jaw shifts, the ball (condyle) will be forced from its normal relationship in the joint, and noise or clicking may occur, as well as compression of sensitive tissues within the joint. The noise or clicking is caused as the ball of the joint slips on and off the cartilage in the joint due to lack of proper bite support.

This noise is measured by a third device called **JVA** (Joint Vibration Analysis), which allows us to analyze the vibrations created in the joint. This gives us insight into the health of the joint. When arthritis has affected the TM joint, the vibrations created develop a higher pitch as the tissues in the joint dry out. This device also allows us to measure improvements in the joint as the sound vibration decreases with the establishment of a more relaxed and stable jaw position.

Technology like this allows for more clarity in the diagnosis and determination of the correct alignment for the jaw. It is objective and repeatable. This leads to more predictable results.

CASE REPORT: This case report is about a 18-year-old woman who was involved in a motor vehicle accident. Her car was struck from the rear. She experienced no direct trauma but did experience immediate head and neck pain as a result of the whiplash. She also experienced clicking in her jaw and restricted opening of her mouth.

An evaluation was done using TENS and a Jaw Tracker. It was observed that the patient's habitual bite was slightly behind and over closed from her more ideal neuromuscular bite position. In other words, the patient had a deep bite that did not give enough support for her joint and jaw muscles.

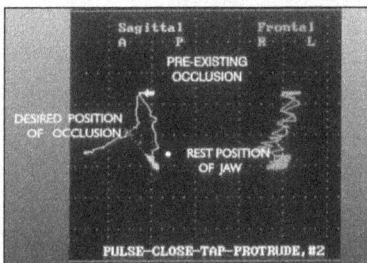

Figure 33: The Patient's bite before treatment for TMJ pain

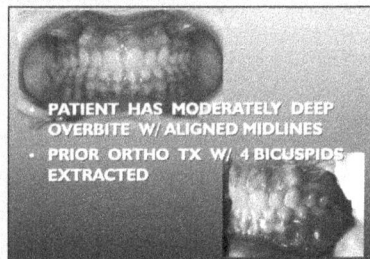

Figure 34: The tracing of jaw movement from a relaxed position to her existing bite and then slide forward depicted on the left.

Joint Vibration Analysis documented the clicking in the left TM joint shown by the sharp peaks in the line at the lower part of the image. The line at the top shows how quiet the right TM joint was.

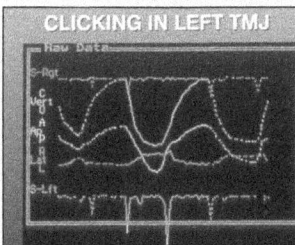

Figure 35: This computer tracing records sound vibrations from the right TMJ (on top) and the left TMJ (on the bottom), with the 3 lines in the middle recording movement in each of 3 planes.

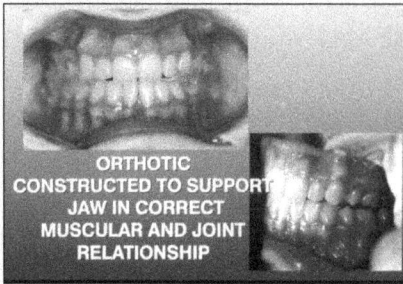

An orthotic was fitted to support the jaw at the neuro-muscular position. Notice that her deep bite appears to be gone with her jaw supported by the orthotic.

Figure 36: Photo showing the patient's bite "raised" with an orthotic on her lower teeth.

Figure 37: This computer tracing compares recordings of sound vibrations from the right TMJ at top and the left TMJ at the bottom, before and after the placement of an orthotic to correct the bite.

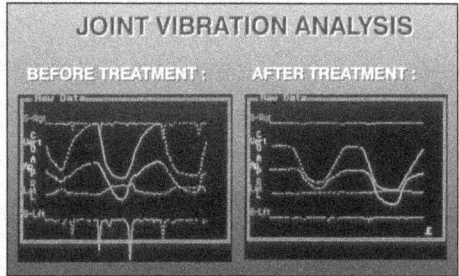

After the orthotic was in place, the patient got more comfortable and her joint became more stable as seen in the image below where there is no longer evidence of clicking in the left TM Joint.

So how do we take these varied concepts and develop an integrative model for dentistry that more completely treats the whole of the patient?

When we evaluate the patient, we need to look at all the factors. There is still a missing link in the consideration of the average dentist who may undertake correction of the bite. That missing link is the rest of the body.

What effect are conditions in the rest of the patient's body having on their jaw muscles and TMJ? What about the effects the bad bite has had on the rest of the body. What kind of compensations may have occurred, resulting in postural misalignments that need to be corrected in conjunction with the dental corrections?

Today, more enlightened dentists are recognizing the need to treat patients with a team approach, to work with a professional trained in the correction of musculoskeletal imbalances such as a chiropractor, osteopath, or a physical therapist.

Because of the vagaries of growth and development, many of us grow up with strain and neuromuscular imbalances within our bodies. As we grow older, we may accumulate the effects of dental care that is less than perfect. Orthodontics may be performed to make teeth appear straight without first determining the proper alignment of the jaw and posture of the body. Broken down or missing teeth may be repaired or replaced without the recreation of an optimal bite. From a practical standpoint, dentistry is often driven by the urgent needs of specific teeth, and all too often, the mouth is not treated as a whole. Over time, there may be cumulative effects leading to a less than ideal bite.

To comprehensively treat the patient, the team needs to consider the following: Does the patient have chronic tightness in their body's myofascial systems?

If so, it needs to be treated. This might be done with acupuncture or using methods of myofascial release, such as those developed by John Barnes, RPT, discussed earlier.

The craniosacral system needs to be brought into balance, often requiring the support of the bite with transitional bite-supporting appliances as corrections are made. This requires treatment by practitioners skilled in methods that originated in osteopathy and chiropractic. These methods are taught in traditional osteopathic manual therapy, craniosacral therapy developed by Upledger, and by the sacral-occipital therapy (also known as SOT) introduced to chiropractic by Dejarnette.

It is common to see that patients with these problems may require low force orthodontic therapies to create symmetry and proper form of the upper jaw, which is attached to the front of the skull, as alignment and balance of the lower jaw are accomplished with the middle and base of the skull.

Many of the patients we see who present for the relief of chronic head, neck, and facial pain related to a bite disorder also have bio-chemical and energetic organ functional disorders that impact their musculoskeletal system. Often there are digestive issues, chronic systemic inflammation (often mislabeled fibromyalgia), and hormonal imbalances. Insight into these may come about by assessment using Applied Kinesiology, an acupuncture energetic evaluation, as well as evaluation from an integrative functional medical physician.

In addition, it is common for us to see problems with misalignment of the bite contributing to narrowed airways that cause snoring and sleep apnea. The resultant poor sleep and associated problems will contribute to the patient's dysfunction and discomfort. This is discussed in Chapter IX: The Mouth and Breathing.

Phasing Treatment

With all of the above considered, the dentist will assist the patient, often in two stages. The first stage (Phase 1) is both diagnostic and therapeutic. First, we need to be clear as to the nature of the patient's problem. Is there a misalignment of the jaw? If so, there are likely cranial-sacral and postural imbalances, too.

What is the condition of the TM joint? Is there displacement of the bony structures and cartilage due to inadequate support of the bite? Has there been a prior injury to the joint with ligamentous strain and loss of integrity in the joint cartilage?

How about the teeth? Are they fitting together properly with the back teeth hitting only on the tops of hills and the bottoms of valleys, without contacts on the slopes? Are the front teeth properly positioned and at the correct angles to guide the unstrained movements of the jaw?

If the alignment of the jaw is off, will the position of the teeth allow the jaw alignment to be corrected without moving them out of the way orthodontically?

Treatment would be provided with removable appliances to provide support and allow for healing of the muscles and strained tissues. This allows for the confirmation of diagnosis before permanent changes are introduced to the bite.

The second stage (Phase 2) of treatment is to make the corrections of the bite permanent. This may involve adjusting the shape of the teeth so they fit better, moving the teeth so they are better aligned, or restoring the teeth to an ideal shape and form so they interact properly in the bite, all along making use of the methods and technologies we have described to ensure the proper outcome.

How to Know If You Have a TMJ Problem

When the TM joint and jaw muscles are not working properly, you may experience any of the following:

- Noise and/or discomfort as you open and close your mouth

- Discomfort in your jaw muscles as you chew and even when at rest

- Ear symptoms (pain, stuffiness or itching, loss of hearing, dizziness, tinnitus)

- Eye symptoms (pain in or behind the eyes, blurring of vision)

- Pain in a tooth or sensitivity of the teeth to cold not related to tooth decay

- Pain anywhere in the face, head, or neck. (It is not uncommon to see people whose only complaint is that they tend to get a stiff neck or recurrent low back pain.)

- Grinding or clenching of the teeth

- Dizziness, or other difficulties standing and walking, unrelated to neurologic disease

In working with patients who exhibit similar symptoms, we will first provide a thorough examination and diagnosis and then will correct these factors applying methods of Dental Somatic Integration, cranio-sacral and myofascial release therapy, acupressure, or acupuncture of reflex points, nutritional therapy, etc.

The muscles of the body are integral to our neuromuscular system and show a correlation between the stomatognathic system and the rest of the body. All of our body's systems are constantly interacting. A healthy bite not only produces a better looking smile but promotes better health and vitality.

CHAPTER VI
How We Know What Is Going On
Methods of Evaluation and Diagnosis

Since the time of Hippocrates, physicians have learned about the nature of a patient's health problem by listening to the patient share the story or history of how their symptoms emerged. In addition, the astute practitioner would pay careful attention to the physical signs apparent as they observed and examined the patient.

In ancient China, the practitioner would also look at the patient's tongue, observing characteristics such as the color and texture of the surface of the tongue for clues about the patient's condition. They would feel the patient's pulses for signs of stress, and over-activity or under-activity of the organ systems. From this, they would develop a diagnosis and plan of treatment, just as acupuncture practitioners do today.

The diagnosis would be based on four separate methods described as:

- Looking
- Hearing (includes smelling)
- Asking
- Feeling

The overall philosophy was that the parts reflected the whole, which led to a holistic health approach. All aspects of the patient may be considered as relevant. In this way, disease was revealed based on a wider array of issues comprising the patient's entire experience.

In the words of Su Ma Qian, a historian of the Han dynasty, "Feeling the pulse, observing the colors, listening to the sounds, and observing the body can reveal where the disease is."

In the west, methods evolved for the microscopic and biochemical evaluation of the body fluids, excretions, and tissues. We culture these same fluids to see if the patient has an infection. We can create images of the internal structures of our bodies with X-rays, MRIs, and ultrasound. Yet still there is much unseen.

In the past fifty years or so, there have been many advances, including a few we will discuss here. These methods give us a unique perspective, allowing us to evaluate changes in the energetic condition of the patient. These methods all have their basis in the principles associated with acupuncture energetics. Given that changes in the function and health of the body's tissues are generally preceded by and associated with changes in the energetic state of that tissue, a method of early screening can highlight when other tests may be indicated and often can help prevent the progression of a diseased state.

These methods can help us assess the potential benefits of different therapeutic agents, as well as the risk in using them, before the patient ingests a medication or supplement. In addition, these methods permit us to find clues to the causative nature of the patient's complaints and can help us to determine what other more conventional testing may be indicated.

The methods I am alluding to are **Electro Acupuncture Diagnosis according to Voll (aka EAV)** and **Applied Kinesiology**.

Electro Acupuncture Diagnosis (AKA EAV) According to Voll

Rheinhold Voll, MD, was a West German physician who developed an interest in acupuncture in the 1950s. In 1958, he combined his knowledge of Acupuncture Energetics with the measurement of fluctuations in the galvanic skin response at acupuncture points. He found, as other researchers have confirmed, that the galvanic skin response was different at acupuncture points as opposed to the surrounding skin. He developed an instrument called the Dermatron to measure these responses.

His device incorporated an ohmmeter that would measure the body's response to a fixed electrical stimulus. When healthy, the response would match the stimulus. In conditions where the tissues associated with the point were inflamed, the response to the stimulus would be exaggerated. When the tissues associated with the point were degenerated, the response would be less than the stimulus.

As he developed his methodology, Voll began to see correlations between the inflamed and degenerative tissues and uncovered that often the patient's dental condition was a factor.

In fact, he found that dental conditions were often contributory to the stress in the body's organ systems and, if unresolved, would impede the responsiveness of the body to his therapy.

When the acupuncture point being tested was connected to a tissue that was in early stages of degeneration, Voll would observe that initially the point would respond to a stimulus triggering a reading on his ohmmeter, but the response would trail off due to the deficient energy being produced in the tissue. He called this phenomenon an indicator drop.

He would stimulate the points with his device to impart energy to the tissue with intention of normalizing it, much as is done with acupuncture needles.

Over 5,000 years ago, the Chinese began to develop a sophisticated understanding of the energetic principles affecting human health, as well as the pathways of energy movement through the body. However, they never defined the energetic connection that each tooth holds to specific meridians. In a matter of a few years, Voll, using his Dermatron, delineated the acupuncture correlations between the teeth and the organ systems of the body. This is shown in the figure below. He was also able to disclose other meridians the Chinese had never defined. If that had been as far as Voll developed his work, it was pretty impressive, but there was more.

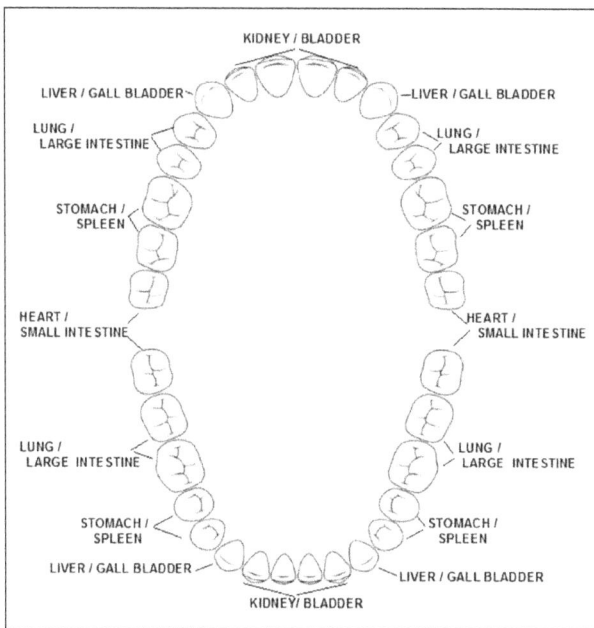

Figure 38: Voll's Dental Meridian Associations

As he continued developing his method, he began to train other physicians. During one such workshop, Voll performed an evaluation of the acupuncture system of one of the doctors in his audience and found that a point that related to the health of the prostate had a strong indicator drop indicating early degenerative changes in the subject's prostate gland. And it was time to break for lunch. Voll announced that after lunch he would continue and demonstrate his treatment of this subject's weakened prostate with electrostimulation of the acupuncture point.

During the break, another doctor in attendance offered the subject with the ailing prostate a homeopathic remedy he said might help with the prostate. The subject put it in his pocket. After lunch, they resumed the demonstration. When Voll re-measured the prostate point, it now tested normal. Voll was puzzled. He was certain about what he had observed before the break. After questioning the subject and finding that he had a prostate remedy in his pocket, it was removed from his pocket and placed on the table. When Voll tested the point again, it revealed an indicator drop just as before. When the subject held the remedy, the indicator drop disappeared. And that is how medication testing with electroacupuncture (aka EAV) according to Voll was born.

Well, how could that be, you might ask. Given the energetic nature of all things and the wondrous nature of our bodies, we are sensitive to the vibes of things around us. In much the same way that we can sense wavelengths of light with our eyes and sound vibrations that pass through the air with our ears, our bodies sense the vibrations emitted from substances that might be either good or bad for us. Most of us do not have conscious awareness of energies, but there are those that do.

Applied Kinesiology

Another great breakthrough came out of the work of George Goodheart, DC. It is called Applied Kinesiology. In 1964, he made an observation while treating a patient that led to the development of a powerful system for diagnosis and treatment based on the testing of muscle reflexes.

As the story goes, Goodheart had a patient who was a deliveryman who complained that he had lost strength in his right arm and couldn't push open a door. Dr. Goodheart had been studying methods developed by physical therapists Kendall and Kendall. They had published a book called *Kinesiology*. They described how to position the limbs of the body to isolate each muscle so that the strength and function of each muscle in the body could best be evaluated.

So here is this guy who can't push open a door. Whenever he attempts to, his shoulder blade comes away from his back and he can't muster the strength. Goodheart quickly finds that the muscle that holds the shoulder blade to the rib cage, known as the serratus anterior, is weak. He positions the patient so that he can push against his hand, as if the patient is pushing against a door and reaches behind the patient to support him as he pushes. By accident, Goodheart had his hand on a point on the fellow's back that resulted in the weakened muscle becoming instantly strong. He took his hand away and the guy's arm weakened again. Then he rubbed the point and the guy's arm got strong and subsequently stayed that way.

As time went on Goodheart began to evaluate the muscle reflexes of his patients more consistently, and drawing from research published by others, he began to see that the integrated function of the muscular system of the body was influenced by the five factors below.

There was potential for (1) disruption of the neural input from misalignments of the spine. In addition, there were (2) reflex points on the body that mediated neurovascular flow to the muscles and (3) neuro-lymphatic drainage of wastes from the muscles. In addition, there was the (4) affects of cerebrospinal fluid flow influenced by the mechanism of the craniosacral system and (5) the influences of the acupuncture meridian system.

One finding that came out of continued research into Applied Kinesiology is that we can find an area of weakness or stress in the body by testing the reflex of a strong muscle. This is done by testing the reflex of a strong muscle while at the same time bringing attention to an area of concern, by having the patient contact this area with their free hand. When we do this, a strong muscle will appear to weaken when we contact the area that is under stress. This is known as therapy localization. Correction of the cause of the problem will result in the muscle that weakened now staying strong when we repeat the test.

In time, it was also found that one could test a subject using Applied Kinesiology to test for sensitivity to substances much like Voll had found with electro acupuncture testing. Using this method, one could readily muscle test for the potential benefit or harm of a food or other substance.

In my work exploring the Dental Connection, I have relied heavily on the principles of Electro Acupuncture Diagnosis and Applied Kinesiology. This integrated approach provides insight into the interactions of the mouth and body. With knowledge of the dental meridian connections, Applied Kinesiology can be used to locate problem areas and show cause and effect relationships, as well as assist in their correction. Understanding the meridians and acupuncture energetics also provide a connection offering insight into the importance of proper jaw, mouth, and tooth alignment.

This has a profound impact on the health and function of all of the body's systems, as was shown by Dr Fonder's research published in the Dental Physician. This was discussed at the beginning of the last chapter.

How we can use Applied Kinesiology and Acupuncture Energetics in dentistry:

- Diagnosis and treatment of TMD

- Diagnosis and mapping of dental somatic reflexes and stress vectors

- Diagnosis and treatment of occlusal stress on an individual tooth

- Dental Somatic Integration

- Diagnosis of fractured teeth

- Diagnosis and treatment of cavitations

- Diagnosis of infections

- Diagnosis of tooth-acupuncture reflexes: differentiating cause and effect

- Materials compatibility testing

- Screening for mercury amalgam field effects

Applying the principles and methods developed through the pioneering work of Dr. Goodheart and Dr. Voll offers a broader perspective on understanding the workings of the human body, as well as expanding our tools for evaluating when things have gone wrong in the body. They both demonstrate functional relationships between the body's parts giving more understanding of the progression of functional disorders and degenerative disease as well as assisting in their cure.

CHAPTER VII
Dental Materials
Interaction with Body Chemistry, Energy, & Function

Materials introduced to the body may be totally inert and cause no effect. They may also lead to toxicity, trigger allergic reactions, or influence the body in other ways that promote a weakness or an irritation. Dental materials can be the cause of all of these adverse responses of the body.

Identifying the possible substances affecting health requires knowledge of toxicity, allergy, and sensitivity combined with an understanding of biochemistry and the electromagnetic nature of the body. Biofeedback methods such as EAV and Applied Kinesiology can help determine an individual's sensitivity to a given material as well as provide information regarding conditions that predispose a person to toxicity and other reactions.

There are also blood tests available that can screen for the likelihood of an individual being sensitive to a given dental material. These are the Clifford Materials Reactivity Tests (http://www.ccrlab.com/) and a similar test available through Biocomp Labs (http://www.biocomplabs.com/index.html).

Toxicity is caused when a material interferes with the body's bio-chemical pathways. This can occur with dental materials used to repair or replace teeth that then degrade in some way giving off molecules of its substance that are absorbed into the internal environment of the body.

Allergic reactions occur when the immune system reacts to a substance. This often occurs immediately although it can also be delayed. It is characterized by the activation of a cascade of events that result in the release of histamine by mast cells and the triggering of inflammation.

There may also be effects that are energetic in nature. The mechanism may be electromagnetic, electrochemical, or still unknown mechanisms.

The most controversial dental material is mercury amalgam used in "silver" fillings. Widely recognized as being poisonous to our entire body, these fillings have been used for many years. The use of these materials is still promoted by the American Dental Association.

In the 1800s, gold foil was used to repair cavities formed by tooth decay. It was an expensive material, affordable only by the wealthy. This changed in the mid-1800s with the development in France of a new material formed by mixing mercury and powdered silver. It was called silver amalgam filling. Initially, its use was resisted by most dentists in America. Those that began to use it could provide care to a greater number people at a more affordable fee than they could with gold foil. Their practices flourished, and over time, more dentists started to use the mercury fillings.

Those that resisted using mercury amalgam fillings did so because mercury was known to be poisonous. The pro-mercury dentists formed an organization that evolved into the American Dental Association. This era has been called the first amalgam war in dentistry. Eventually, most dentists were using mercury amalgam fillings, and it continues to be widely used to this day.

The second amalgam war began when chemist Alfred Stock again raised concerns in 1926. His research defined "micromerculialism," a toxicity disease from low-level chronic exposure, and he recognized that dental fillings were a significant source of mercury exposure. His research was ignored. In 1931, another chemist reported finding traces of mercury in urine and fecal matter after fillings were put in. However, the need for inexpensive dental materials outweighed any outcry.[20]

Finally, in 1973 after evaluating the evidence, Brazilian Olympio Pinto, DDS, introduced Hal Huggins, DDS, from Colorado to the work he had done investigating the harmful effects of mercury. Dr. Huggins became convinced that the mercury did leak and was harmful to patients.

Dr. Huggins became an outspoken crusader and took on the American Dental Association. After authorities revoked his license to practice dentistry, Huggins earned a master's degree in immunology and toxicology. He then collaborated in the development of blood tests to assess the biocompatibility of dental materials in general. These are the blood tests now offered by Clifford Labs and Biocomp mentioned earlier.

Huggins found that most lab tests were variable in their ability to disclose mercury toxicity as the cause of a patient's complaint. "There is no one single test that determines if a patient is or is not mercury toxic. The reason for this is that mercury attacks <u>all</u> tissues, not just one place. Genetics will determine where that attack will focus, and chemistry can point to the direction of the battle."

In 1984, The International Academy of Oral Medicine and Toxicity (IAOMT) was founded to document and promote new science on safety of dental materials and techniques.

This resulted in a surge of research by scientists and clinicians leading to improved information about toxicity and oral health.

---

20. Alfred Stock, 'Dangerousness of Mercury Vapor', 1926, http://iaomt.org/alfred-stock-1926-dangerousness-mercury-vapor/.

Some findings of this research included:

- Mercury has different forms. In the human, gut bacteria can interact with it and convert it to a more toxic form.

- Mercury creates problems by altering the biochemistry of the body.

- Mercury has a strong affinity for sulfur. Due to this, mercury will bind with sulfur found in proteins, enzymes, etc. This results in changes that keep them from working properly. It can affect the processes that help us in the conversion of the energy of our food into the form of energy used by the body: ATP.

The questions raised about mercury amalgam causing health problems have met opposition from those claiming that there was no evidence of mercury causing a specific disease. And that is the crux of the problem. Heavy metal toxicity caused by mercury and other metals like lead are often contributory to multiple disease conditions.

As we have discussed, new perspectives are emerging on the multifactorial cause of chronic degenerative disease. Toxins like mercury can be subtle in their effect, leading to changes in the competency and efficiency of different biochemical pathways within the body, slowly causing changes over time. Such changes may be written off as aging when in fact they are not. Progressive physicians practicing integrative medicine recognize that heavy metal toxicity is a common denominator impairing the body's healing and will routinely screen for it.

An interesting note about mercury amalgam fillings is their impact energetically within our energy body. In every patient we have examined, it has been observed that the presence of mercury amalgam fillings creates suppression energetically within the acupuncture meridian of Stomach. This is readily demonstrated using Applied Kinesiology. In treating patients, we see that the removal of the last bit of amalgam in the teeth on one side of the mouth results in strengthening of the Stomach meridian on that side. We call this a field effect, reflecting the innate sensitivity of our bodies to a substance that is harmful.

What You Need to Know If You Choose to Have Your Mercury Fillings Replaced

Mercury amalgam fillings must be replaced with carefully selected bio-compatible alternatives. Because there is mercury released as a vapor when these fillings are removed, specially developed protocols, including an oxygen mask, dental dam, and vacuum are used to minimize your risk of exposure.

Once the mercury fillings have been removed, a cocktail of vitamin C, activated charcoal, and chlorella is ingested to facilitate chelation and excretion of any mercury that manages to pass the protective barrier.

If you choose to eliminate mercury fillings from your mouth as a step toward improving your health, it is important to prepare your body

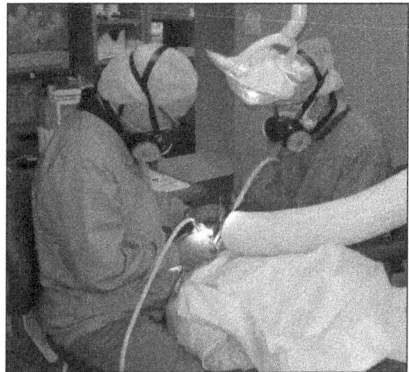

Figure 39: Mercury-Safe removal protocol established by the IAOMT

properly to maximize the potential health benefits. Preparing your body to rid itself of heavy metals always begins with proper nutrition.

The following guidelines aid in the body's detoxification:

- Eat a diet high in organic vegetables and fruit. Limit, if not eliminate, the consumption of fish and fish products during detoxification. (They may contain mercury. Larger fish such as tuna and swordfish, being higher on the food chain, will have higher levels of mercury.)

- Drink plenty of water every day. Adequate water is necessary for the proper functioning of routes of detoxification and excretion.

- Study of the function of the body and the literature on natural healing reveals there is an order to things in the body. The bowel, kidneys, and sweat glands of the skin are the major route for mercury elimination from the body.

- Good blood and lymph circulation are necessary for the transport of toxic substances in their passage out of the body. The liver needs to be functioning well, being the major organ for screening toxins from the blood and labeling them for excretion from the body.

- Exercise is important to keep all your organs working properly.

- It is very important that your body can rid itself of the toxins. If constipation is a problem for you, try a natural colon cleansing product to improve bowel function. Consider eliminating gluten and dairy from your diet.

**MERCURY TOXICITY CAN ONLY BE DIAGNOSED
AND TREATED BY A LICENSED PHYSICIAN.**

Important Aspects of a Mercury Detoxification Program

Mercury causes problems within the body because of its ability to create a toxic condition at very low levels of exposure. The chemistry of mercury is such that it develops strong attractions for sulfur-containing compounds within the body (enzymes, hormones, proteins, membranes, etc.), and then alters the ability of these compounds to perform their supporting role in the symphony of our body's biochemistry. In binding to these sulfur-containing compounds, mercury displaces other elements such as selenium, zinc, magnesium, and manganese. These elements are crucial to facilitate the action and efficiencies of biochemical interactions. Because the mercury displaces them, their concentrations unbound in the body become elevated and they are excreted, ultimately resulting in deficiencies.

Huggins was one of the first to report on the need to load the body with trace minerals as part of a detoxification protocol. In severe cases, it is probably best to assess the body for deficiencies of trace elements. Imbalances that are present can be targeted. In most individuals, it may be more practical to offer the body a supplement that provides a general base of minerals such as BodyBio electrolytes.

Sulfur compounds are good cellular and intracellular chelators. Compounds that are used medically for heavy metal chelation take advantage of mercury's strong attraction for sulfur. Commonly used agents include DMPS (sodium salt of 2,3-di-mercapto-1-propanesulfonicacid also known as Dimaval) and DMSA (meso-2,3-dimercaptosuccinic acid). Both have been well researched, with DMPS being considered more effective than DMSA.

A word of caution with DMSA. It has been suggested that DMSA affects the permeability of the blood-brain barrier, making it useful to pull mercury from the brain. However, if the connective tissue concentration in the body of Hg is greater than in the central nervous system, use of DMSA can lead to Hg migrating into the brain. Perhaps this is the cause of a transient "brain fog" reported by some who have used DMSA for mercury detox. It is also recognized that use of the sulfur-containing amino acids, methionine and cysteine (as NAC) can also be helpful.

Another compound frequently used by physicians is EDTA (ethylene diamine tetraacetic acid). It is great for chelating lead and other common heavy metals, though does not contain sulfur and therefore is not as effective for chelating mercury.

Another sulfur-containing compound that is being recommended by many physicians as an adjunct to mercury detox is MSM (methyl-sulphonyl-methane). For a natural source of sulfur, raw garlic and supplements that are garlic derivatives are known to be helpful adjuncts.

Chlorophyll containing compounds from plants are helpful, too. Chlorophyll is a naturally occurring compound with a strong ability for binding metal. From a chemical perspective, it is similar to our hemoglobin molecule that binds iron. These types of chemical compounds are called porphyrins. Porphyrin-based supplements such as Biotecs Research Porphyra-Zyme are considered helpful to pull mercury from the connective tissue and the gut.

Chlorella is an algae that can act as a natural sponge for pulling mercury from the gut. It is important that the source of chlorella being used is certified free of mercury or other heavy metal contamination (*Biosorption of Heavy Metals*, Bohumil & Volesky).

Cilantro tincture (Dragon River Herbals) has proven itself an effective herbal adjunct for heavy metal detoxification. Omura's work established cilantro (coriander) as an effective herbal chelator that pulls Hg from nerve tissue into connective tissue. It should be followed by a chelator like DMPS, or other sulfur-rich compounds that will pull from connective tissue and facilitate its transport for excretion. Cilantro can assist in the removal of mercury out of the brain. It is eliminated while the person exhales (stand back). Some caution should be exercised in use of cilantro before comprehensive routes of excretion are established.

Vitamin C and its role in detoxification: the ubiquitous vitamin C plays a role in so many aspects of the body's metabolism and structural support. Its role in supporting the body's detoxification pathways is undisputed. As part of a well-rounded program, vitamin C should be used both before and after removal of amalgam fillings to aid in mercury detoxification. It can be used in high dosages in the range of

5-10,000 mg a day (adjust the dose to bowel tolerance), though should be discontinued for 24 hours before dental visits because it does interfere with the benefits of local anesthetics.

Activated charcoal and bentonite clays: they strongly absorb mercury and other toxins. In addition, there are a number of different vitamin, herbal, and homeopathic treatments available from herbalists, homeopaths, physicians, and other healthcare practitioners to help detoxify patients from mercury poisoning.

If you suspect you may have symptoms caused by mercury toxicity, you should consult with a licensed physician who is experienced in the diagnosis and treatment of heavy metal toxicity.

Other Commonly Used Dental Materials Are Cause for Concern As Well

Mercury amalgam is not the only material used in dentistry that poses a risk to our health. For many years, plastic fillings, also known as composite, have provided a tooth-colored material used in the repair of both the front teeth and the back ones. The plastics have also been used as dental sealants to protect against decay forming in the deep grooves and fissures on the surfaces of the back teeth.

These materials had been based on the chemistry of a compound known as BPA (also known as Bis-GMA, Bis Phenol, etc.) These materials were first developed in the 1930s and have been used in many consumer products as well as eventually being used in bondable fillings beginning in the 1970s. Early on, there was controversy about their use as it was known that BPA acted as an estrogen mimicker.

An estrogen mimicker will cause a response in the body as if estrogen is present even when it is not. BPA does that because a part of its molecular structure resembles a part of the estrogen molecule, and it is able to interact with estrogen-binding sites in our body's cells. In a sense, it fits like a key in a lock designed to be opened only by estrogen. In recent years, there has been a grassroots effort to get manufacturers to stop using BPA in their products. This has resulted in changes.

Being in the habit of screening patients for compatibility of the materials we use, we have observed that some of the plastic filling materials still being used appear to cause reactions energetically similar to those that had been known to contain BPA.

It appears that in an effort to improve, some dental manufacturers have re-engineered the BPA compound, allowing them to call it something else. Unfortunately, it appears that some of these plastics still retain an estrogen mimicking property.

We now have safer choices for healthy fillings and dental appliances. There are composite fillings on the market that were never based on BPA and are thought to be safer. Improvements in ceramic, porcelain, and other materials have provided better options and combinations to suit specialized needs.

Gold, the oldest dental material, is still given preference because of its strength, durability, and gentleness on neighboring teeth. The potential problem is that gold is always used in a blended alloy with other metals so that it is not too soft. Often gold may be mixed with palladium in dental alloys. This makes the final result harder. The problem is that palladium has the potential to trigger allergic and toxic reactions. When screening materials, we rarely see a patient who responds favorably to gold alloys with palladium. In those that do, the gold content is generally 85% of the total content of the alloy.

Dental implants have introduced another area of concern for biocompatibility. Initially, pure titanium was used. However, due to limited experience and poor design, there were structural failures that led some manufacturers to correct the underlying design issues and others to use titanium alloy with aluminum and vanadium.

Most people that we screen with kinesiologic muscle response testing respond poorly to the implants made with titanium alloy with aluminum and vanadium and seem to be okay with pure titanium. European manufacturers, especially those from Germany and Switzerland, are using pure titanium. In recent years, implants made from a material called zirconium have been introduced.

Benefits of Pure Titanium Implants

- They have a long track record of results.

- Titanium implants are made in two parts. The part that goes below the gum can be covered when the implant is placed to provide undisturbed healing. The part that goes above the gum to hold the tooth can be screwed into place later, and the shape is readily customized to adapt to the requirements of the bite or for cosmetics.

- Pure titanium is one of the most biocompatible metals with long use in orthopedic medicine.

- Titanium implants encourage an intimate adhesion of bone around them that makes them suitable for the long-term replacement of teeth.

For some time, we used only pure titanium implants because we found that most patients were not sensitive to pure titanium. Now we are able to offer implants made of a material called zirconium that is metal free.

Benefits of Metal-Free Zirconium Implants

- Zirconium has become popular as a desirable implant material because it interacts well with the natural gum and bone, making it biocompatible.

- Metal-free implants are biological dental implants, meaning they're a more holistic option for those interested in treatments that support total health.

- For cosmetic reasons, zirconium is a better choice. Titanium dental implants may cause a dark line around the gum. Zirconium is a more natural color, eliminating this effect.

- When it comes to dental hygiene, zirconium is favored by many periodontists because it discourages the buildup of plaque and tartar in a way that titanium does not. That means less risk of gum disease in the future.

- Because of the increased interest in holistic dentistry and metal-free treatments, zirconium dental implants are gaining in popularity. For patients who suffer from sensitivity to titanium, metal-free dental implants offer an excellent alternative.

CASE REPORT: Sonia came to us about seven months after she had received two implants replacing teeth in her upper right jaw. Almost immediately after they were placed, she didn't feel right. A week after the placement of the implants she got a rash on her face. The dentist gave her antibiotics, though that did not help. She developed a burning sensation in her tongue and stiffness in her neck.

She told us that her lips became prone to swell and then the skin on her lips would peel. She became sensitive to makeup. Applying any would cause her face to swell and the skin would redden. She had become emotionally stressed due to the prolonged discomfort and uncertainty of the future.

When we performed muscle reflex testing, her strong arm would weaken when we touched the area around the implants. In addition, she would weaken when we touched along the associated meridians, both along the Large Intestine meridian along her arm as well as the Stomach and Spleen meridians running down the front of her body.

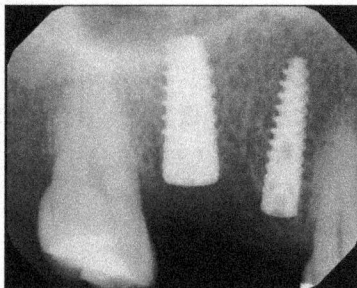

Figure 40: The appearance of these implants on the X-ray image was unremarkable.

Upon research to determine the composition, we found that these implants were made of a commonly used titanium alloy that used aluminum and vanadium, often written as 'Ti-6Al-4V' and called Grade V (5) titanium. Grade IV (4) titanium is pure titanium.

Sonia consented for us to remove the implants. We had concern that since the implants had been in almost seven months the bone would have healed in intimate contact with the implant surface making removal quite difficult. We studied the case carefully and planned for all contingencies, acquiring an array of special instruments that might become necessary.

On the day of surgery, we flapped back the gum and saw that the bone had grown partially over the top of the implants. Upon seeing this, I expected that the removal might be quite difficult. Once we had carefully removed the bone from the top of the implants and removed the small cover screws sealing the top of the implants, we were able to fit special wrenches to apply force to unscrew the implants from the bone. To my surprise, they came out quite readily. Due to her sensitivity to the materials, her bone had not been able to form intimate contact with the implant surface. The rest of the procedure was routine and uneventful as we grafted bone and sutured the area. Sonia was overcome with a sense of relief, grateful that her ordeal had finally come to an end.

Recognizing how dental materials impact and affect overall health and acknowledging that certain individuals may react differently to a specific material necessitates that patients be screened on an individual basis for the materials to be used. Applied Kinesiology is a simple and practical means of doing this. Blood tests for material compatibility may also be used. The best results will come in a sensitive individual from the use of both methods.

CHAPTER VIII

Focal Infection

A Challenge to the Immune System & the Bioenergy Field of the Body

---

"It falls upon the dentist and oral surgeon to study the diseased conditions of the mouth ... The next great step in medical progress in the line of preventive medicine should be made by the dentists. The question is will they do it."

—Charles H. Mayo, MD of the famed Mayo Clinic.

As discussed in an earlier chapter, the teeth are connected by the meridians to all parts of the body. As a consequence, stress or disease within a tooth will influence other regions of the body and vice versa. This is readily demonstrated by means of kinesiologic reflex testing and electroacupuncture diagnosis.

When the teeth are diseased or stressed and acting as an influence elsewhere in the body, they are defined as being a *focus* of irritation within the energy systems of the body. The most common condition of a tooth that results in it acting as a focus is when the tooth has become infected because of a degenerative condition of the nerve pupal tissue that often results in root canal treatment of the tooth.

Frequently, root canal treated teeth will act as persistent foci despite the appearance of a successful root canal treatment. This is not a new concept.

Root Canal Treatment and Biological Dentistry

The benefit of having root canal therapy (RCT) preformed is to preserve the tooth if an infection or inflammation has compromised it. This aids in the maintenance of the structural integrity of the mouth. The technology of treatment has advanced dramatically over the past ten years and continues to advance.

The tooth is first isolated, and then the dentist opens the tooth by drilling a hole on the top of the tooth and removing the infected pulp inside the canal. (One to four canals can be present depending on position of the tooth in the mouth.) The canals are filled, and then a filling material or crown is placed to seal the tooth.

However, there are concerns being raised about the potential negative influences associated with teeth that have been treated. The concerns are based upon the potential for teeth to become toxic, and a source of biochemical and energetic disturbances within the body. Is the problem caused by root canal treatment, where the patient can have a reaction to materials used to disinfect and/ or fill the canals of the tooth, as some have suggested, or is it due to contaminants introduced into a tooth by the disease process that are not eliminated by RCT?

I feel that both can play a role in the success or failure in the outcome of a root canal treated tooth.

It has been common practice in many dental offices to use toxic chemicals (cresatin, formocresol) for disinfection of diseased teeth, though this practice has gradually declined. We have seen patients whose infected teeth had been treated with these toxic materials end up with chronic issues of an overactive immune system. These chemicals are similar to those used to turn trees into telephone poles. They are often called fixatives, as they interact with biological molecules, especially proteins, and alter them, rendering them inert. They have a strong odor and are capable of permeating beyond the site where they are placed. This means when placed in a tooth, they will leak beyond the tooth, affecting the tissues surrounding them and rendering them as foreign to our body. Teeth that are treated this way most certainly end up becoming a focal irritant.

Another problem with treatment lies with poor technique. If the root canal system is not adequately cleaned or not adequately sealed, this will also lead to failure.

Even with competent treatment, there is always risk of a tooth becoming re-infected. This was illustrated by research where virgin non-diseased teeth were to be extracted to make room for orthodontic care, and the patient (dental students) agreed to have the tooth root canal treated some months before the tooth was to be extracted for the purpose of the study. Even in teeth that had been disease-free before treatment, bacteria were found in the fine lateral canals of the teeth after treatment and in the tissues surrounding the roots.

Dr. Lerner's View

In my experience, many root canal treated teeth appear to be without negative influence. But not all are, and that requires us to consider all factors when recommending treatment. Root canal therapy properly performed with materials that are biocompatible for the individual can be a valuable service allowing for the preservation of a tooth.

The best methods available today utilize lasers such as the Biolase Waterlase and ozone treatment for the most thorough sterilization of the root possible. By avoiding the extraction of teeth with degenerated nerves, we are able to prevent other situations (e.g., structural imbalances, alterations to other teeth for holding bridges, the need to place implants).

When a root canal treated tooth is found to be creating a disturbance to the rest of the body, it can sometimes be corrected by retreatment of the root canal. However, careful consideration must be given to extraction of the tooth. Long standing infection leads to a chemical change of the tooth's root, and the tooth becomes a foreign body, triggering reactions of the immune system. Such teeth must be extracted because they are now toxic to the body. Each root canal tooth should be tested individually for its effect on the rest of the body.

Does the Diet of the Patient Have an Influence on the Prognosis?

Diets high in sugar and starches can promote a biological terrain that supports the growth of fungi and yeast in the body, such as seen in Candidiasis. Such a condition can promote a higher incidence of fungal issues in dead teeth, whether treated with root canal therapy or not.

The Evidence about the Systemic Consequences of Toxic Teeth

The potential for a tooth to be an agent in the development of disease was first discovered by Dr. Weston Price in the 1930s. His research involved extracted teeth that were infected and toxic being placed under the skin of rabbits. He found that:

- These teeth implanted led to disease that mimicked the disease of the human tooth donor.

- Vital healthy teeth implanted led to no disease.

This was widely accepted at the time as many physicians saw their patients' health improve after the removal of infected teeth. The Mayo Clinic embraced this philosophy. They based their recommendations on the Focal Infection Theory.

In time, perhaps partly due to Flexner's influence on medicine, the Focal Infection Theory fell into disfavor as the fields of medicine and dentistry made efforts to be more scientific and had no understanding of the mechanisms involved.

Today physicians around the world engaged in biological medicine find that extraction of root canal teeth contributes to improvement in many medically compromised patients. Reasons why this can occur are suggested below.

We now understand more about the immune system and its capacity to be overactive as seen in many autoimmune conditions. Teeth that still harbor infection or are embedded with the toxic byproduct of infections, or toxic chemicals introduced into a tooth by a dentist treating an infection are acting as a foreign body and over stimulating the immune system. Bioenergy testing (kinesiology/electroacupuncture) reveals that some root canal teeth are reactive in some patients. The issue appears to be complex.

Dead teeth and teeth with degenerated pulp tissues that have not yet been treated with root canal therapy always demonstrate evidence of causing an electromagnetic field disturbance in the body. This is evident when evaluating teeth via bioenergy testing. There will be evidence of a disturbance at the tooth, as well as at acupuncture points on associated meridians.

Teeth with diseased and inflamed pulps causing toothache will trigger reaction with the autonomic nervous system that is reflected in activation of acupuncture points within the ear that are readily detected with bioenergy testing.

What Influences Are Seen with Dead Teeth— Whether Treated by Root Canal Treatment or Not?

When performing bioenergy evaluations using kinesiology (muscle response testing), a disturbance being caused is evidenced by a strong muscle going weak when the tooth in question is touched. Such a response is often evident even if we just bring our probe (or finger) close to the tooth (i.e., in its energy field).

Once the tooth (or teeth) is identified, the patient's general energetic status is examined as discussed in the section on Applied Kinesiology.

Once we have a determination of the patient's energetic state, we can temporarily switch off the weakening reflex associated with the tooth by rubbing the skin overlying it softly in the direction of the patient's feet. Then test the tooth again. It will seem to test strong. Now evaluate the patient again. Areas of disturbance that are a direct effect of the tooth will also disappear temporarily.

When the tooth is retreated, these areas must also clear. If they aren't, the likelihood is that the tooth is still a disturbance and extraction should be considered. When infected teeth are extracted and the tooth socket thoroughly cleaned, the meridian associated with the tooth will test clear. If it doesn't, then we aren't done cleaning out the diseased tissue from the socket. More thorough cleaning will resolve the disturbance within the meridian. We then apply ozone gas to the socket for sterilization of anything that might persist.

What Are the Energetic Influences Associated with Extracted Teeth That Had Shown Disturbance in the Body?

In our clinical studies, what we are seeing is that after we extract a toxic tooth, the patient's energy field will improve, with the strengthening evident where there had previously been a weakness. Interestingly, if we then have the patient hold their extracted tooth, the energetic disturbance that was evident in their body will seem to return as long as they hold the tooth. This continues to occur with toxic teeth even if they have been passed through a steam autoclave to render them sterile.

This phenomenon occurs even when these sterilized toxic donor teeth are energetically evaluated with other individuals. Consistently, the individual being tested will demonstrate the same patterns of energetic disturbance that had been associated with this toxic tooth when it was still present in the mouth of the donor. This is consistent with the findings from Weston Price's research with rabbits many years ago. Teeth that have become toxic contain toxic agents that contribute to degenerative disease.

An example of the effects of a toxic tooth on the acupuncture meridians is provided in the following case. When the patient had first been seen, we evaluated the tooth that had root canal treatment by means of Applied Kinesiology muscle testing and found a weakness in the tooth. We suggested at the time that the patient have the root canal recleaned and sealed. He declined treatment.

A year later, he complained to me that he was having problems with his ankle on the same side. He asked if it might be affected by the tooth that I had raised concern about. I pulled out my manual on Applied Kinesiology to determine how I could directly test the muscles in his ankle. We found that two muscles on the inner part of the ankle were weak. Both of these muscles were on the Kidney meridian, the same meridian that passed through the tooth. The tooth still caused a strong muscle in his shoulder (the Deltoid) to weaken when we tested. He agreed for me to reclean and re-treat the tooth.

As we proceeded, I checked the muscles in his ankle again as I recleaned the tooth, and they were immediately testing at normal strength. The problem in his ankle resolved and did not reoccur.

I suspect that along the way he had strained his ankle and the problem in the meridian caused by the tooth interfered with the healing of the muscles. He had received physical therapy, acupuncture, and chiropractic treatment without resolution until the problematic tooth was identified and resolved.

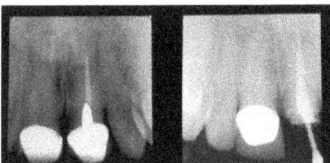

Figure 41: The tooth before re-treatment on the left and after on the right.

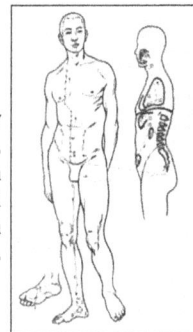

Figure 42: The Kidney Meridian, the link between the front teeth and the muscles in the ankle.

117

How Does a Tooth Become Toxic?

The most common cause of the dental pulp becoming degenerative is caused by the process of tooth decay progressing to the point of invading the pulp tissue (live tissue in the tooth). This then permits bacteria to have a direct pathway into the tooth. The process of inflammation and infection of the pulpal and then the periapical tissues (around the root tip) will lead to the generation of many toxic chemicals. These include volatile sulfur compounds, hydrogen sulfide (H_2S), and methyl mercaptan (CH_3SH), as well as other compounds. If a tooth is not treated in a timely fashion, the tooth will likely become so toxic that it should not be treated but extracted.

How Do We Know If a Tooth Is Toxic and Should Be Extracted?

In dentistry, we have relied on the appearance of the tooth and surrounding tissues on X-ray. A limitation is that a conventional X-ray will not always clearly show us when there are changes in the bone at the tip of the root indicating an abscess is forming. This is illustrated in the case that follows.

On the next page is a conventional X-ray showing two teeth that had root canal therapy performed years before. The patient complained of persistent discomfort on and off for years. The area had been evaluated by a few dentists over time, yet none had ever found evidence of a problem. When we muscle tested the teeth as described previously, the patient's strong arm (testing the deltoid muscle) weakened, giving evidence of a problem.

A second X-ray was taken. This one, a dental cone beam provided a three-dimensional view. A darkened area representing disease around the root of the tooth is clearly visible. Extraction of the tooth resolved the patient's complaint.

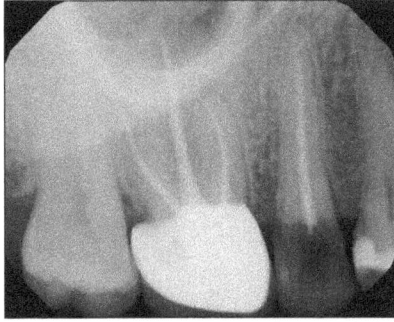

Figure 43: Conventional X-ray did not show the problem.

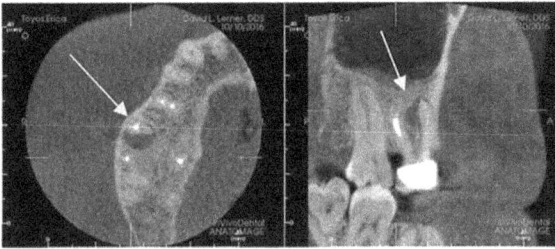

Figure 44: A cone beam image allowed us to view the tooth from different perspectives. Now we could see the darkened area around the diseased tooth.

One of the world's leading practitioners of biological medicine is Dr. Thomas Rau from the Paracelsus Clinic in Switzerland. He describes his approach to healthcare and his view of root canal treated teeth.

"Here at Paracelsus, we take a very different approach, relying instead on our ability to reinvigorate the body's own life forces, which include its ability to heal and regenerate. We call this practice 'Biological Medicine.' Its methods arise from the distinct medical tradition of Switzerland and southern Germany, which in the 500 years since the experiments of the original Paracelsus have evolved a more holistic and natural science of health."

"80% of women seen in Paracelsus clinic with diagnosis of breast cancer have a toxic root canal treated tooth on the meridian that passes through the breast."

So again, the question may be asked:

How do we know if a root canal treated tooth is toxic and should be extracted?

Some biologically trained physicians and dentists would say, "Always."

I believe it depends on the situation. I have seen numerous elderly and relatively healthy patients with root canal treated teeth that showed no evidence of toxicity or systemic influence. However, I have also seen many patients of all ages and levels of health where infected or toxic root canal treated teeth were demonstrating signs of toxicity.

I believe there are a number of variables to be considered:

- How infected had the tooth been prior to treatment?

- How long had it gone untreated?

- How thoroughly and competently was it cleaned and sealed by the dentist?

- Were there toxic compounds used in the process of treatment?

- Were more advanced methods, such as a laser or ozone, used in the process of disinfection of the tooth?

- What about the health, constitution, and diet of the patient?

An infected or toxic root canal treated tooth should be extracted in a patient with compromised health when it is demonstrated to be acting as a focal stressor affecting the associated meridian and therefore having a systemic affect.

The bottom line is that the patient deserves the right to make an informed decision about the treatment they choose, understanding the risks and long-term consequences.

CHAPTER IX
The Mouth and Breathing

The form of the mouth and the bite can make breathing easy or more difficult. The airway is unrestricted and free of tension when there is proper development of the mouth and face. However, it can be affected by physical strain in utero, at birth, and during early development.

Birth trauma can cause strains in the myofascia of the cranial cervical area with resultant tension of muscles and distortion in the balance and symmetry of the skull. In newborns, this can interfere with normal function of suckling, creating difficulty for the infant to latch on to the breast. Extended difficulty can cause the development of imbalanced muscles of the lips, tongue, jaw, and throat.

With under development of the lower jaw, it will tend to be receded creating an overbite. Because the jaw has not grown forward, it will tend to constrain the area of the throat thus narrowing the airway. As a consequence, the tongue loses its reference to the developing space in the mouth and fails to conform and push against the roof of the mouth. This action is essential for the development of the palate and upper jaw as well as influencing the growth of the facial bones. The child might become a mouth breather.

If an infant experiences the world as an unsafe place, there will be disruption in the patterned development of the nervous system particularly involving the function of the cranial nerves.

An infant fed with a bottle and artificial rubber nipple may have difficulty developing and maintaining balanced muscle tone and coordinated reflexes during swallowing due to the resistance created by the material the nipple is made of. When breastfed, the soft and pliant nipple of the mother's breast will yield to the forces of the tongue and promote better development of the orofacial muscles. In addition, if the flow from the artificial nipple is too fast, the infant may be overwhelmed and develop guarding reflexes with their tongue in an effort to protect their airway.

Consumption of improper food that is not natural can result in development of allergies and congestion of the nasal pathways. This encourages the development of mouth breathing, which deprives the infant and young child of the beneficial effects of breathing through their nose. Air passing over the fine hairs within the nose results in warming and moisturizing air breathed in as well as stimulating the production of nitric oxide, a chemical essential in regulation of endothelial tone of our blood vessels. With mouth breathing this benefit is lost.

The habits developed can persist throughout life. Accidents, improper dental work, and other conditions can cause or exacerbate problems with the mouth later in life as well, which can bring on breathing problems in adulthood.

Snoring and Sleep Apnea

The most common breathing complaint in adults (or their sleeping partners) is snoring. The vibrations of the soft tissues of the upper airway produce noises we call snoring. Often the snorer does not even know it is happening, and some people adamantly refuse to believe they snore. The narrower the airway space, the louder or more frequent snoring will be.

Sometimes snoring is more than noise. In general, it is a sign that there is an unbalance in the system. Snoring can be a sleep disturber, and it can be a sign of more troubling problems. It can be a symptom of a more severe disorder, sleep apnea.

Sleep apnea occurs when the tongue and soft palate collapse onto the back of the throat, blocking the upper airway and causing airflow to stop. The oxygen level in the body drops low enough to move the brain out of sleep and partially awaken itself. Then after gasping for breath to get the airflow going again, the body moves back into deep sleep. This dangerous and detrimental cycle plays out and repeats itself over and over again, all night long.

Low oxygen levels and interrupted sleep create all kinds of new potential problems. People who have sleep apnea often do not have a high level of overall health. As well as exhibiting general un-wellness, sleep apnea patients often have higher risk of heart disease, hypertension, strokes, and accidents.

Sleep apnea is diagnosed based on measurements recorded during an overnight sleep study that is analyzed in coordination with the patient. Some treatments include:

- **Good sleep habits** – healthy balanced sleep with regular hours

- **Weight loss and exercise** – whole health approach with clean eating. Reducing the circumference of the neck associated with weight loss will reduce the tendency for the airway to be blocked

- **Continuous positive airway pressure (CPAP)** – a mask that delivers air through a tube

- **Oral appliance therapy** – a custom fit oral mechanism that is worn during sleep

An oral appliance designed to support the jaw in a relaxed and unstrained position during sleep can help support an open airway between the base of the tongue and the throat.

Oral appliances work best for snoring and mild-to-moderate sleep apnea. These small, comfortable devices are similar to orthodontic retainers or sports mouthguards.

Approximately 40 different appliance designs have been approved by the FDA for the treatment of snoring and/or Obstructive Sleep Apnea (OSA). Oral appliances may be used alone or in combination with other means of treating OSA, including general healthcare, weight management, or CPAP. Oral appliances work in several ways:

- They reposition the lower jaw, tongue, soft palate, and uvula.

- They stabilize the lower jaw and tongue.

- They increase the muscle tone of the tongue.

Many dentists have the required training in oral airway issues and breathing problems, and can help you discover your best treatment option. Having a holistic professional who can see the bigger picture will often provide a source of relief and comfort in dealing with these conditions.

CHAPTER X
The Body, Mind, and Mouth
as Thought and Emotion

A human being is an organized and intelligent field of energy. The organization of our energy begins with the fusing of the sperm and egg from which we came. On a physical plane, we can see the body as a tissue that has different composition and form in different regions. There is what we know as skin, with connective tissue, bone, and other differentiated tissue below. We see arms and legs and ears and eyes and our mouth. All different aspects of the whole.

Through the tissues of our body, we experience life and emotion. Different emotions are specific in the nature of the sensations they create in different parts of our body. We might think of emotion as 'energy in **motion**'. In the healing traditions of China, mental and emotional issues that would arise would be treated by getting the Chi (energy) of the patient moving again.

A healthy and integrated human being has balanced function and freedom of movement in a non-toxic state with emotional equilibrium. Being posturally balanced with connective tissues free of restriction is a goal to strive for, as well as a system free of chronic toxicity and inflammation. Balanced chemistry and stress-free function of all body systems, including balanced function of our brain with an open mind and clarity of our thoughts are also requisite for optimal health.

This blend of mind, body, and spirit opens the pathway for disciplined living and the evolution of a higher level of consciousness. All of this effectively encourages knowledge, wisdom, longevity, and a balanced life.

This is the basis for healing traditions from around the world including yoga. In the yogic tradition, the body is seen as having different energy centers or chakras. Each chakra is involved in different aspects of our emotional and spiritual experience.

The throat chakra that includes the jaw and mouth influences our ability to communicate and self-express. When the throat chakra is blocked or out of balance, there will be interference with energy flow, with both physical and emotional signs.

The physical signs may be tension or pain in the jaw (TMJ), neck, or shoulders, as well as headaches and a propensity to ailments of the throat and larynx[21].

In addition to physical signs of chronic blockage in the throat chakra, there is possible emotional, psychological, and spiritual impact as well.

There may be a fear of speaking, a difficulty in expressing thoughts, shyness, inconsistency in speech and actions, social anxiety, inhibited creativity, stubbornness, and/or detachment [22].

Because of the structural and biophysical interactions within the body and

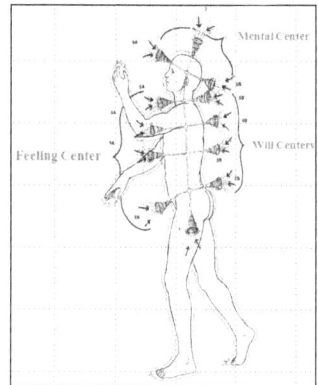

Figure 45: The Chakra Energy Centers of Ayurveda

21. 'Throat Chakra Blockage', http://www.chakras.info/throat-chakra-blockage/.
22. Ibid.

particularly within the craniosacral and myofascial meridian systems, physical constraints and imbalances of force in the patient's bite
and jaws will influence the energetics of all of the chakras. Thus, the
patient's experience of the movement of energy (emotion) in their body
will impact their perceptions of self (psychological) and how they relate
to the world around them. Our self-image and sense of identity are
influenced by our mouth, as are the comfort and ease with which we
are able to express ourselves in speaking and with facial expression.

Those patients who have gone through a process of Dental Somatic
Integration report that they not only feel more relaxed and comfortable with their mouth, but more at ease within their body. Often they
will say they feel more grounded, as indeed they are, both physically
and energetically. As the mouth is brought into balance so is the spine
and pelvic girdle. The improved flow through the myofascial meridians
allows for better continuity and flow of the electromagnetic forces of
the earth below and the heavens above through the body.

CASE REPORT: Some years ago, we treated a lady for jaw clenching
who had also been diagnosed with multiple sclerosis. We fitted her
with an upper appliance that allowed only her lower front teeth to touch
the appliance, preventing her back teeth from colliding against sloping
surfaces. (Remember back teeth should only touch on tops of hills and
bottoms of valleys.)

Shortly after she started to wear the appliance, she shared that she had
suffered from chronic depression that was alleviated when she wore
the appliance. By using Applied Kinesiology, I found that when the appliance was not in her mouth there was myofascial constraint within her
neck, shoulder girdle, and upper chest that disappeared when the appliance was in her mouth. Her depression was being caused by a physical
constraint on the flow of energy between her head and chest and the
rest of her body. Her throat chakra had been blocked.

Clearly, there may be multiple causes of depression. Deep sadness brought about by the loss of a loved one, the loss of a job, or a sudden change in life circumstance may bring on a state of depression, known as situational depression. Also, it has become widely known that bio-chemical imbalances as well as disruptions of proper brain chemistry triggered by food sensitivities or exposure to toxic chemicals can bring about depression.

It is important to be aware that for many, depression may represent a state of blocked energy flow, often brought about by poor structural support of the jaw and improper fit of the bite.

The Human Organism Is a Manifestation of Energy

Wilhelm Reich, MD, studied lifelong behavioral patterns in individuals with psycho-spiritual trauma early in life. He believed that the individual's personality and character were shaped by the chronic holding onto of protective reflexes long after the threat had disappeared.

His insight into the potential for the development of "armoring" within the myofascial systems of the body in response to perceived psychic traumas inspired him to conceive a method for freeing the individual from its effects. He did this through a rigorous process of physically challenging their defenses to break them down. Ultimately, the individual experiencing these defenses would then experience their bodies in a relaxed state. Reich viewed the mouth and throat as one of the primary areas of the body where energy would be blocked.

When the flow of energy is blocked at the mouth and throat, the health effects can be significant. As we have seen, in early years, growth and development can be stunted. All of the connecting meridians and energy centers are affected. When the teeth, mouth, jaw, and connected tissues and structures are properly aligned and correctly developed, a healthy posture develops providing an open flow of energy throughout the body.

Our Connections to All That Is

We have spoken about the use of Applied Kinesiology to give us feedback and insights into the workings of the body. Psychiatrist Dr. David Hawkins takes this one step further in his book *Power vs. Force: An Anatomy of Consciousness.* In the book, he describes how he used Applied Kinesiology to determine the true answer to all questions he might pose by tapping into universal consciousnesses.

> "The individual human mind is like a computer terminal connected to a giant database. The database is collective human consciousness itself, of which our own consciousness is merely an individual expression, but with its roots in the common consciousness of all mankind.
>
> This database is the realm of genius; because to be human is to participate in the database, everyone, by virtue of their birth, has access to genius. The unlimited information contained in the database has now been shown to be readily available to anyone in a few seconds, at any time and in any place. This is indeed an astonishing discovery, bearing the power to change lives, both individually and collectively, to a degree never yet anticipated." [23]

From this, we can take an understanding of the mind-body to project (think of visualization) energy fields that are healthy and life supporting. In a sense, our beliefs create our map of realty, which can become fixtures in our mind, then cause us to project into our energy field an image that then becomes self-fulfilling. It is through our belief and intent that we can promote healing, or disease.

We can steer clear of destructive patterns. Inside our consciousness is the ability to connect with our central nervous system and stimulate, adjust, or tweak any inconsistencies blocking the healthy flow of

---

23. https://universeisathought.files.wordpress.com/2014/11/power-vs-force-hawkins-david-r.pdf.

energy. In this way, we can promote relief from a health condition as our mind-body connection imprints a remedy.

Years ago, another way of saying this was shared by a friend, Dr. Ann Carpenter. She once said to me, "Ayurveda (the ancient healing tradition of India) views the process of healing as the body remembering its identity."

Another example of the body-mind as an energy field is demonstrated in the work of Mark Seem, L.Ac., the founder of Tri-State College of Traditional Chinese *Acupuncture. He* developed a model of acupuncture that seeks to bring the body in balance with its energetic blueprint. His book, *Acupuncture Imaging - Perceiving the Energy Pathways of the Body,* describes the potential and benefits of working to bring the body-mind to its highest level of integration and function by recreating the body-mind as a true depiction of its genetic potential, free of restrictions, compensations, and imbalances imposed by maladaptive responses to social, psychological, and physical stressors.[24]

Acupuncture can free a patient's body from the effects of psychic and emotional trauma, and reactions to the tensions of the world. This permits new patterns to be formed. In this type of energetic therapy, the acupuncture facilitates a more fulfilling sense of being in their body-mind connection, providing deeper healing for the patient.

The following case study illustrates the mind-body connection from a dental perspective.

CASE STUDY: A patient of ours was referred for the extraction of her wisdom teeth. A few weeks after the oral surgeon had dismissed her from follow-up care, she was still experiencing some tenderness in the lower left jaw and an aggravation of a chronic headache condition.

---

24. Mark Seem, PhD *Acupuncture Imaging: Perceiving the Energy Pathways of the Body* (Healing Arts Press, 2004).

Examination revealed tenderness still present over the site of extraction of the lower left wisdom tooth. Evaluation utilizing Applied Kinesiology revealed a blockage of lymphatic flow from the jaw as well as weakness energetically along the associated meridian. We applied acupuncture magnets to encourage the flow of energy.

Upon her next visit two weeks later, she reported that her pain had lessened with the magnets, but had worsened again after she removed them. The pain worsened for two to three days at which point she had a dream in her sleep of a doctor visiting her and performing some vague treatment. When she awoke, the pain was gone and did not return.

What is interesting is that the pain worsened until she had this dream of the doctor treating her. In a sense, it is as if our treatment with the magnets provided a temporary imprint of a state of restored balance for the body that, once it faded, was restored with more permanency by recalling it in a dream. The mind-body has to reestablish a connection and then the symptoms dissipate.

The mouth is where thought becomes speech so it is understandable that it is one of the crucial locations for mind-body wellness.

CHAPTER XI
Healing Through Holistic Dental Medicine

"If I needed to remove either the medical or dental component of my clinic, I would keep the dental because chronic problems will not resolve without biological dental care."

- Dr. Thomas Rau, Director of Paracelsus Clinic, Switzerland

We have discussed different connections between your mouth and the rest of your body. This has been just an introduction and represents our understanding of these relationships at the time of writing these words. We keep learning new information every day through our own experience and the experience of colleagues from around the world.

I would encourage educating yourself and seeking health practitioners with whom you share a common philosophy. We all must be our own healers, though often we cannot accomplish it on our own.

To summarize there are different dental risk factors that can be an influence on our health. They are:

Dental caries or tooth decay that can lead to breakdown of tooth structure and infection of the tooth. Dental caries primary cause is to be found in an improper diet that changes the biochemistry of saliva and promotes the growth of decay causing bacteria such as Strep Mutans.

Once a tooth becomes infected attempting to preserve the tooth with root canal therapy can lead to systemic risks of chronic exposure to toxins created by the waste products of the bacteria persisting in the roots. I have seen many patients where there was clear evidence that their root canal teeth were toxic and having a negative consequence on their health.

Periodontal disease is not just a localized condition of the mouth but will often have systemic consequences. The bacteria involved with causing inflammation of the gums and breakdown of the supporting bone will get into the blood stream and are linked to numerous systemic health conditions including stroke and cardiovascular disease, cancer; especially pancreatic cancer, arthritis,.....

The materials conventionally used in dentistry to repair or replace teeth often involve metals or plastics that have the potential to trigger reactions in the immune system, can cause toxicity as in the case of mercury amalgams, or act as endocrine disruptors as has been seen with the use of composite fillings that contain Bis-Phenol (aka BPA).

Proper development of the jaw structures and a good bite promote good stress-free alignment within the musculo-skeletal system. Poor development, improper treatment of crooked teeth and malocclusion, or improper repair and replacement of missing teeth can compromise the bite further causing stress throughout the body leading to chronic pain and other symptoms. Taking a whole body approach is essential both to the diagnosis and treatment of these conditions.

These problems in jaw alignment are also recognized as a major cause of snoring and sleep apnea due to the impingement created on the airway from our nose and mouth to the lungs. Dental correction can pen the airway, improving breathing and leading to improved vitality.

We hold a vision for the future of health care in which the dental profession plays a central role as guardians of the well being of our patients. Central to this new paradigm is the philosophy of prevention that has been a hallmark of the dental profession since Dr. G.V. Black, a pioneer in the dental profession. An essential aspect of our role is as both educator and facilitator to empower our patients in making informed choices that may improve their health and quality of life.

Traditional dentistry and medicine are rooted in a legacy of great technologic advancement and service in the relief of suffering associated with disease. We have been quite successful. Yet, despite all our advances in technology there is an increase in morbidity from chronic degenerative disease, and healthcare costs continue to climb.

It is my contention that we are limited by holding to an outdated disease oriented paradigm. We are still influenced by the constraints imposed in medical-dental education almost one hundred years ago by the Flexner Report which sought to exclude from the medical (dental) paradigm disciplines not then understood by the chemical and surgical sciences of the day.

In the past century the explosion of knowledge in all of the basic and life sciences has been profound. The development of quantum physics and an understanding of the fundamental energetic nature of (cellular and molecular) biology have been revealed.

The challenge of Dentistry is that our perspective is not yet broad enough. We seek to comprehend the truth, yet are limited by our belief systems. This document is my humble attempt to assist in the process of removing those blinders.

The tissues of the mouth; the teeth, jaw bones, the gums, the bite, the muscles, and the Temporomandibular joints exist within a continuum that is both structural, biochemical, and bioenergetic in nature. The mouth will both reflect changes in the health of the whole body, as well as, be the cause or contributing factor to dysfunction and disease elsewhere.

The body is an integrated whole, there are no separate systems.

My intention has been to share information that has not only given me a different view of dentistry, but of life itself. It is my hope that understanding the Dental Connection will give you a new and broader perspective as well.

ADDENDUMS

Chapter 2 Extras

My Paradigm

by David L. Lerner, DDS, P.C., C.Ac., F.I.N.D.

Biophysics: field theory and quantum physics, the energetic nature of all things, electromagnetic fields of the body, role in development and differentiation, holographic nature of the body, resonance phenomenon, homeopathy, the science of acupuncture, tooth-meridian associations. Implications for dentistry.

Biochemistry: the energetic nature of biochemistry, concept of Biologic Terrain, qualities of water, nutrition and degenerative dental disease, the relationship of digestion (beginning with mastication) and assimilation, disorders of immune function, disorders of mineral metabolism and pH in dental caries and periodontal disease, toxicology and detox pathways, inflammation and hyper-immune states, dental toxicology, and materials biocompatibility. The field effect in biocompatibility. Implications for dentistry.

Biomechanics: Structure and function, tensegrity (the balance of tension and compression that generates structural integrity), connective tissue and the myofascial kinetic pathways, craniosacral, neuromuscular, Applied Kinesiology, occlusion, plane of occlusion, vectors of force, the periodontal ligament, neuromuscular reflexes and proprioception, the physio-pathology of functional disorders. Opportunities and challenges in restorative and orthodontic therapy.

Chapter 3 Extras

The Dental Connection in Cardiac Pain and Arrhythmia

by David L. Lerner, DDS, P.C., F.I.N.D., C.Ac.

In her work on the study of trigger points, Janet Travel, MD, spoke of her observations that trigger points in the pectoralis major muscle seemed to generate reflexive reaction in the heart resulting in irregular heart-beats.[1] Sometimes the pain originating in the tight tender areas of this muscle were perceived by the patient as coming from their heart.

Pectoralis Major Muscle & the Cardiac Trigger Point Phenomena

A) overlapping referred pain patterns of two parasternal trigger points (x's), located in the medial sternal section of the muscle

B) location of the "cardiac arrhythmia" trigger point (x) below the lower border of the fifth rib in the vertical line that lies midway between the sternal margin and the nipple line. On this line the sixth rib is found at the level of the tip of the xiphoid process (arrow)

This vertical line corresponds to the pathway of the Kidney Meridian and the trigger points are found at K21, 22.

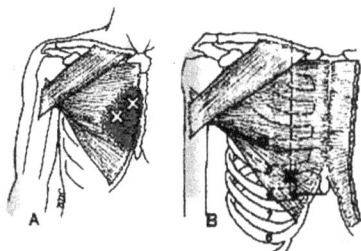

Figure 46: From Travell & Simons'
Myofascial Pain & Dysfunction:
The Trigger Point Manual
Used with permission from the publisher

Other authors have spoken of the relationships between dysfunction of the pectoralis major and associations with cardiac dysfunction.

Schwartz and Bourassa[2] state that in the Coronary Artery Surgery Study Registry of the 1970s, normal angiograms were found in 19% of patients, and they suggest that the statistics today are not much different. They raise the question: "Is there a non-cardiac cause of chest pain?" and list numerous possible causes including chest pain of musculoskeletal origin.

In an article entitled "Cardiac Pain Syndrome,"[3] Andrei Pikalov, MD, Ph.D., writes about three variations of anterior chest wall syndrome (ACWS) that are associated with cervical, thoracic, and cervical-and-thoracic pathology. All three variations involve muscular pain, dystonia, dystrophy, and neurovascular changes in the pectoralis major and other tissues of the anterior chest wall.

In an article entitled "Chest Wall Syndrome: a common cause of unexplained cardiac pain," Epstein et al.[4] describe twelve cases with severe, often incapacitating chest pain initially believed to be cardiac in origin. All twelve were shown on subsequent evaluation to have chest wall syndrome. Diagnosis was confirmed by chest wall tenderness simulating the spontaneously occurring pain in all. Seven patients had chest wall syndrome in conjunction with other associated cardiac conditions. Five patients had isolated chest wall syndrome with no cardiac disease.

Further associations have been written about in the acupuncture literature. Mark Seem, Ph.D., writes about what he calls the state of cardiac alarm as a final stage in a progression of chronic stress and fatigue through four stages that he describes in his book *Acupuncture Physical Medicine*.[5] He describes patients suffering from tightness and constriction in the chest with shallow breathing and a tendency to hyperventilate. Often these patients were "experiencing anxiety, sometimes feelings of impending doom." He described these patients as often having symptoms of "pelvic collapse" with tightness in the muscles on the side or front of the lower abdomen. He further describes a band of tightness in the pectoralis major muscle involving tightness at acupuncture points K22, St18, and Per19. He describes this condition as capable of mimicking a heart attack, leading patients to the cardiologist or emergency room.

So, what is the Dental Connection here? Well, it is rather interesting, as we shall explain. Dysfunction of the pectoralis major muscle appears to frequently be associated with a primary dental problem.

The bite of the teeth plays a very important and central role in maintaining symmetry and balance throughout the muscular system of the body, as we shall describe below. When the bite is off balance, it will result in changes throughout the body, weakening pathways through the muscular system that follow the course of the acupuncture myofascial meridians. There will also be disruption to the autonomic nervous system that controls the automatic functions of the body including our breath, heart rate variability, and digestive function.[6]

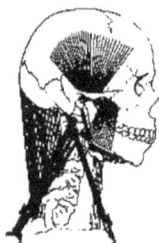

Figure 47: The muscles connecting the jaw play a role in posture of the head and neck.

The jaw muscles, directly supported and influenced by the bite, are in intimate association to the rest of the muscles of the head, neck, and shoulder girdle. Changes in the bite will directly affect these muscles, sometimes increasing the tension of a muscle, sometimes interfering with the muscles ability to do its job.

The ability of muscles to function normally can readily be evaluated using the methods of Applied Kinesiology, developed by chiropractor George Goodheart. His work drew heavily on the work of Kendall and Kendall, physical therapists who wrote a description of methods to evaluate the strength and competency of most of the major muscles of the body.

Goodheart found that when weak muscles were present, they could often be strengthened by specific improvements in nutrition, correction of specific cranial or vertebral misalignments, and stimulation of appropriate acupuncture points.

By applying his methods in the evaluation of disorders of the bite, we are able to demonstrate the relationship between different aspects of the patient's anatomy and physiology.

As we examine patients for systemic influence of their bite imbalance, we have seen numerous patterns of dysfunction. For now, we shall focus on the patterns we see associated with dysfunction of the pectoralis major muscle and the heart meridian.

As a result of deficiencies in the height of the bite and misalignment of the jaws, the muscles on the side of the jaw, the masseter and temporalis, will not work properly. There will be a tendency for these muscles to over contract. When this happens, the next muscle in the postural chain, namely the sternocleidomastoid, will be disrupted, and there will be a loss of normal muscle tonus. This results in instability of the collarbone and, in turn, affects the pectoralis major. This will be evident when the strength of the pectoralis muscle is evaluated using basic muscle testing as described by Kendall and Kendall, shown below.

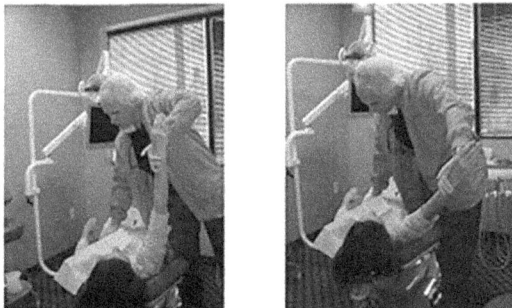

Figure 48: On the left, the doctor challenging the strength of the pectoralis major muscle; and on the right, the muscle had no strength and yielded indicating a disruption to its function.

Further evaluation using Applied Kinesiology may be performed utilizing the phenomenon of therapy localization as developed by Goodheart and described by Walther.[7] When this is done, a strong muscle, such as the middle deltoid, is challenged, and then with a free hand, the clinician can contact a point or region of the body. If there is a disruption of physiology in the underlying tissue, the muscle that was previously strong may be observed to lose its capacity to maintain a sustained contraction and immobilization of the associated limb. In other words, it will appear to weaken.

When this is done in patients with bite imbalances, and contact is made with the masseter muscle as the patient clenches their teeth, the strong muscle (middle deltoid) will appear to weaken in most instances. If the sternocleidomastoid muscle is contacted, a similar phenomenon may be observed. If the pectoralis is contacted along its lateral border, again the strong muscle (middle deltoid) will weaken.

When contact is made along the myofascial pathway of the Heart meridian in these cases the strong indicator muscle (middle deltoid) will be seen to weaken. In all cases where we have seen this pattern), we will also find that there is a disruption to the Kidney meridian on the patient's opposite side. This is most evident if contact is made with acupuncture point K3 on the medial aspect of the foot above the arch.

Now if we find the pectoralis muscle to be weak in the chest and touch the Kidney 3 point on the opposite side which we therapy-localized as above, we will find that the weak pectoralis muscle will strengthen. The same will occur if an acupuncture needle is placed in the Kidney 3 point; that is, the previously weak pectoralis muscle will get strong. However, in most cases observed, this phenomenon is short lived because once the patient bites down, the pattern of muscle dysfunction is generated again and the pectoralis muscle is weak.

The only way to permanently correct the dysfunction of the pectoralis muscle is to restore balance to the involved jaw muscles using first an orthotic (appliance) for temporary support and then permanent correction of the patient's bite. When this has been done, symptoms of anxiety and heart rhythm irregularity have resolved. In summary, many patients experience symptoms for which there is no apparent cause. This is true with some patients who report symptoms of anxiety and cardiac arrhythmia. To better understand the causal chain involved, we need to be able to see the patient as a whole through the perspective gained from interdisciplinary study and exchange of ideas.

David L. Lerner, DDS, P.C., C.Ac., F.I.N.D.
2649 Strang Blvd, Suite 201
Yorktown Heights, NY 10598
info@holisticdentist.com
914-245-4041

Endnotes

1. J.G. Travell 1 and D.G.Simmons, *Myofascial Pain and Dysfunction; The Trigger Point Manual*, (Williams and Wilkins, 1983).

2. Leonard Schwartz, MD; Martial G. Bourassa, MD , 'Evaluation of Patients With Chest Pain and Normal Coronary Angiograms' *Arch Intern Med.* (2001) 161:1825-1833.

3. Andrei Pikalov, MD, PhD, 'Cardiac Pain Syndrome', *Dynamic Chiropractic* 11/4 (1996), Vol. 14, Issue 23.

4. S. E. Epstein, L. H. Gerber and J. S. Borer, 'Chest wall syndrome. A common cause of unexplained cardiac pain', *JAMA* (June 29, 1979) Vol. 241 No. 26.

5. Mark D. Seem, Ph.D., *Acupuncture Physical Medicine; an Acupuncture Touchpoint Approach to Chronic Fatigue, Pain, and Stress Disorders*, (Blue Poppy Press, 2000).

6. Aelred Fonder, D.D.S., *The Dental Physician*, (University Publications, 1977).

7. Applied Kinesiology.

www.ingramcontent.com/pod-product-compliance
Lightning Source LLC
Chambersburg PA
CBHW031941190326
41519CB00007B/609